My Boy Butch

My Boy Butch

The heart-warming true story of a little
dog who made life worth living again

Jenni Murray

HarperCollins*Publishers*

HarperCollins*Publishers*
77–85 Fulham Palace Road,
Hammersmith, London W6 8JB

www.harpercollins.co.uk

First published by HarperCollins*Publishers* 2011

1 3 5 7 9 10 8 6 4 2

A catalogue record of this book is
available from the British Library

ISBN 978-0-00-736220-2

Printed and bound in Great Britain by
Clays Ltd, St Ives plc

Mixed Sources
Product group from well-managed
forests and other controlled sources
www.fsc.org Cert no. SW-COC-001806
© 1996 Forest Stewardship Council

FSC is a non-profit international organisation established to promote the
responsible management of the world's forests. Products carrying the FSC
label are independently certified to assure consumers that they come
from forests that are managed to meet the social, economic and
ecological needs of present and future generations.

Find out more about HarperCollins and the environment at
www.harpercollins.co.uk/green

For David, thanks for finally saying, 'Yes.' J.

Contents

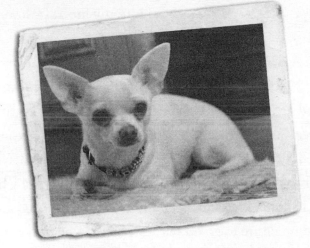

Introduction

As I sit here writing, he is curled up amidst a pile of cushions behind me on the bed. He appears to be asleep but he isn't. He is alive to my every sound and movement. If I make as if to get up, one eye will open, peer out from inside his cocoon and he'll leap into instant wakefulness and energy. He will follow me everywhere. He is, the family jokes, my shadow.

This book is about the dog who changed my life. It's about a Chihuahua, the smallest of dogs with the

biggest of hearts, who came into my life at its lowest
ebb.

A diagnosis of breast cancer had been confirmed
on 20 December 2006. It was the day my mother
died after a long battle with the cruelly debilitating
effects of Parkinson's Disease. Quite how we struggled through Christmas I shall never know. My
father suffered the immeasurable grief of a man who
had adored the same woman for almost 60 years and
had no desire to go on without her. He needed every
ounce of energy I could muster. I had to face a
mastectomy between Christmas and New Year,
organise my mother's funeral and then begin a course
of chemotherapy which would last for half the year.

In the midst of the exhausting effects of the treatment – as I tried to keep the rest of the family, my
two sons, Edward and Charlie, and my partner,
David, in some semblance of normality and sanity –
my father succumbed to lung cancer in June. Thus,
within a few short months, I, an only child, lost the
parents who had always been a reliable rock throughout my life, faced the possibility of my own demise,
had to accept that my children were now grown up

and becoming increasingly independent, and that my partner was in as great a state of shock as I was.

He and I would rattle around the family home, which now seemed over-large and silent. I grieved for my parents and my health. He too was full of sadness. We had been together for almost thirty years, so my parents were family to him as they were to me and my children. But the greatest pressure, in the aftermath of all this sorrow, was a doom-laden sense that we were now the older generation; that we would be next to face the draining deterioration that ageing brings, and we were uncertain that doctors who predicted a good prognosis for me were telling us the truth.

It seemed that any plans for a fulfilling and energetic middle to old age might be scuppered by my illness; and David, who had never known me to be anything but a cheery livewire, constantly occupied by home, children, work and friends, suffered an unspoken terror that he, like my father, might be consigned early in the middle years of his life to caring for a sick woman or, even worse, might lose her altogether. The days passed heavily.

And then came Butch. His name is not altogether incongruous. He may be a mere Chihuahua, but he has the heart and stomach of the fiercest Rottweiler, and when we stay in the Wuthering Depths of my London basement flat on the days I'm in the capital for work I no longer fear the night-time intruder, knowing he will warn me of any impending danger.

Butch began to replace tales of my children in the weekly newsletter that I write online for the BBC. He has become the star of the show, receiving presents – he always wears his gift of a black leather collar with the diamante inscription 'BAD BOY', confirming that he's joined his mistress as a gay icon – and regular enquiries as to his health and his latest antics.

At the literary festivals I have attended over the past months to publicise my last book, *Memoirs of a Not So Dutiful Daughter*, the first question is frequently, 'How's Butch? Why didn't you bring him with you?'

I am, I fear, upstaged, even in his absence!

His youth, verve and uncritical, unconditional devotion have made me look forward to getting up in the morning – food, a walk, a game in the garden and to coming home – no longer to an empty house, but to a smiling and enthusiastic welcome.

He is an affectionate, devoted and sometimes hilarious companion. He has made life worth living.

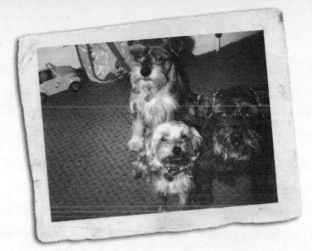

Chapter One

A Dog Is for Life

There was always a dog. If not real, then imagined. I don't precisely recall at what stage it began to dawn on me that the most powerless creatures on the planet seemed to be little girls, but I can't have been much more than a toddler when I developed a deep resentment of being bossed about. It had quickly become apparent that I was considered fair game for parents, grandparents, disapproving aunts and the gang of local big boys who tittered at any valiant attempt to join in with climbing a tree, kicking a ball or steering a tricycle. They made it quite plain they would as soon drown in the dirty duckpond as be seen actually playing with a creature that jabbered incessantly and sported (generally unwillingly) a ribbon in its hair.

But a dog, I knew – partly by instinct, partly from the books my mother read to me – would never snigger or criticise or make demands. It would revel in your company and obey the most peremptory of barked orders. 'Sit, heel, stay, roll over' would be music to its ears. It would fetch the ball you were doomed to play with alone. Should you find yourself being beaten up by the biggest bully on the street – a not uncommon occurrence – it would tear out his throat in your defence. Should burglars dare to enter at the dead of night, it would rip out the seat of their pants and hold them, terrified, until the constabulary turned up.

In my vivid, infantile imagination I dubbed myself 'the mistress' and ceased to be some pathetic, undersized weakling, expected to sit nicely, knees demurely together with neatly brushed hair and scrubbed apple cheeks.

At night, after the bedtime story, I dreamt that a heroic Shadow the Sheepdog lay snoring at the end of my bed as I slept or Lassie traversed the known universe to be at my side or Timmy and I strode about solving crimes and saving damsels in distress.

I begged and pleaded with my mother for a dog of my own. She was adamant that she had quite enough to do, thank you very much, with a house, a child and a husband to run around after. Why would she need the responsibility of a dog?

'I know full well,' she'd say, 'that you'll tell me you'll look after it. But you won't. I'll be left to walk it, feed it, and I'll be hoovering all day to get rid of its hairs.'

My mother was obsessively houseproud and, although I doubt she realised it at the time, had indeed articulated one of the first lessons in the canon of feminist commandments:

'Thou shalt not buy any animal you are not prepared to clean up after. Men and small children have a tendency to lie about their readiness to attend to such matters.'

Thus the lonely existence of an only child continued until the happy coincidence of two not entirely
unconnected events. The first involved my disappearance. I was four. This was the 1950s and, apart from
reading, listening to the wireless and being helpful
around the house, there was not much to keep a child
entertained at home.

Parents were relatively unconcerned about their
youngsters playing out. In fact, for a mother whose
work was staying home, cooking, cleaning, washing
and ironing, it was something of a relief to have her
offspring out from under her feet for an hour or two.
There was none of today's dire warnings of stranger
danger, nor were there enough cars on the road for
incessant traffic to be seen as much of a threat. There
must have been a degree of parental concern as I was
frequently warned not to 'go off'. 'Stay in the garden
or the fields or the street where I can keep an eye on
you.'

Only, on the day of my disappearance, I was
George – the best fictional role-model any growing
girl could have and the star of my favourite Famous
Five books by Enid Blyton. How I longed to have a

name that could be made to sound like a boy's, to show scant interest in the making of cakes and sandwiches and be the protagonist in whatever adventure I could conjure. Naturally, at my heel, would be the celebrated Timmy. I don't recall that Timmy was ever held on a lead in the books, he simply ran along obediently by George's side.

But I knew, whilst still a tiny girl, that even slow-moving traffic could cause devastation. A small boy, the son of a neighbour, had been killed not long before whilst playing under the Co-op grocery van. He'd been crushed as it pulled away and all of us who were used to playing in the street had seen the white, drawn faces of the mothers who comforted the one who had lost her child.

We had stood at our kitchen windows as the cortège with the tiny coffin had driven slowly down the road and had sobbed in sympathy with our own parents. I know now that people would think it silly to compare the threat to an imaginary dog with that of an all-too-real child, but to me, at my young age, the danger was genuine. I was so worried that during our long trip looking for thrills in the village Timmy might run into the road, I had his leash clutched in my hand.

We were gone for hours. We popped into the Co-op store and trailed our feet through the sawdust on the wooden floor, sniffing the pungent aroma of freshly ground coffee and watching the man in the white coat and cap slicing through the huge smelly cheeses with an enormous wire – scary, just like a guillotine. Then he'd cut through a ham with a whirring circular saw, leaning over the counter and asking whether my dog might like a taste. We said thank you, I scoffed the lot and we left and crossed the street to Tom the fruit and veg man who'd been kind enough to return a lost and beloved teddy I'd once left behind. He too welcomed Timmy and me and offered an apple. I declined, explaining that the dog wasn't keen on fruit and I mustn't as it was nearly teatime. We set off home, climbing the steep hill, tired by now, and hungry.

For years my mother would describe in exacting detail the moment she saw her diminutive daughter come at last into view, dragging a piece of string behind her and demanding, imperiously, 'Come along, Timmy, don't dawdle. We'll be in terrible trouble if we're late for tea.' Until I had my own children, I never understood why mothers, who are hugely relieved at seeing their child safe and sound after long, anxious hours, shout, scream and are furious rather than huggy, kissy and nice. Very cross was what she was. Timmy and I were sent upstairs to my room in disgrace and with no tea. I think she must have sat in the kitchen thinking how much more sensible it would be, should I ever dare to disappear again, for me to be accompanied by a real dog who might provide some protection rather than by a useless figment of my imagination.

Which is when we had the visit from Cousin Winnie. She shared my mother's Christian name and her penchant for upward mobility. She bred corgis with a pedigree as long as your arm in tacit emulation of the Royal Family. She had a problem. Her prize bitch had shown scant regard for the preservation of the blueness of her blood and had indulged in illicit relations with some mongrel mutt from the wrong side of the tracks. The resultant puppies were far from pure bred. She was having trouble getting rid of them and just wondered if we might be prepared to take one off her hands.

Thus, on my fifth birthday, I came down to breakfast and was given a parcel of irregular shape to open. It contained a collar and lead. The lead had a tag on which was engraved, not Timmy, but Taffy. A minor disappointment, but an acceptable nod in the direction of his half Welshness, and my parents led me by the hand, trembling with anticipation, to the shed outside.

There, lying nervously in a far from comfy plastic bed (easy to keep clean, said my mother; he won't be in it for a minute, thought I, he'll be snuggled up on my blankets) was everything I'd imagined Timmy/ Taffy to be. Gingery brown, huge, meltingly dark eyes, stiffly pointed ears, spindly legs and the longest, waggiest tail I could have hoped for. The mongrel genes had won out big time over the short-legged, stocky corgi. He hopped out of the bed, wriggled over to where I crouched on the ground and licked my hand. I knew I would never be lonely again.

Taffy turned out to be the fulfilment of every one of my childish canine fantasies. He was a willing and uncomplaining accomplice in any silly adventure in which I chose to involve him, mostly concerning the tracking down of evil criminals hiding out in the woods near the house – he did the sniffing – or unearthing buried treasure in the garden. He did the digging, much to my father's displeasure when the only things of any value we managed to uncover were the seed potatoes he'd put his back out planting. If there was trouble as a result of our adventures we'd simply escape to my bedroom and dig out an Enid Blyton for further inspiration.

We spent hours together strolling around the cemetery. It may seem strange that a young child should be fascinated by death, but I found it all quite touching. On days when it was too wet or cold to visit the graves I would read the notices in the *Barnsley Chronicle* and found the often trite poetic clichés utterly beautiful.

In the burial ground itself, which was a short stroll from our front door, there were long, carefully tended paths to walk along and then pause at the poor, simple headstones of those without much money and the grandiose mausoleums, almost like houses, that were the final resting place of the rich merchants and coalmine owners of the past.

We'd take a few sandwiches and a bottle of pop and sit by the elaborate gravestones of tiny children who'd died in the 1800s. There were Sarahs and Edwards, Pollys and Williams. In some families four or five babies had survived for only a few months and I would read the unbearably sad poems out loud to Taffy, ears cocked, ever attentive as the tears poured down my cheeks.

'With angel's wings she soared on high, To meet her saviour in the sky' is the only one that sticks in my memory, apart from the scary one on a grown-up's grave positioned near the great wrought-iron gates at the entrance and which I copied into my diary.

Remember well as you go by,
As you are now, so once was I.
As I am now so shall you be.
Prepare yourself to follow me.

I never failed to read it as we passed the grave and never failed to be absolutely terrified by it. We would run home to the warmth and safety of my mother's kitchen and her wasted words of advice.

'Of course you're not going to die. They didn't have such good doctors in those days. And if it upsets you so much, don't go there.' But for most of our walks I was irresistibly drawn to what Dad always tried to make me laugh by calling 'the dead centre of Barnsley'. Not funny. Not funny at all.

An alternative route was the lane opposite my grandmother's house which led to a bridge over the railway line and then the river. We would pause on the bridge and wait for a train to pass, the steam puffing up and over us. I loved it and the promise of bigger and better places it offered. Taffy hated it and would cower at my feet until the roaring noise was well past. But he loved the river. He swam and rolled around in the muddy banks whilst I paddled in the shallow water, dipping a fishing net in among the weeds and bringing out tiddlers and sticklebacks.

I had a jam jar with string tied around the neck for ease of carrying and at the end of the afternoon we'd carry our prize home to my mother's 'Don't bring that smelly jar in here, and keep that dog outside – he's filthy.' We both had to hover around by the back door, whatever the weather, until she found time to turn on the hosepipe and give him a shivering wash down. He leapt at the warm, dry towel I proffered – old and tattered and kept for the job – and revelled in a good rub down.

I learned a lot from Taffy. As I grew older and struggled with the inevitable anxieties and tensions of the teenage years, he became my confidant when I realised that secrets told to a dumb animal were much less likely to be passed on than if they were told to someone you'd thought you could trust as a friend.

I discovered that kindness, low-voiced firmness and bribery tend to achieve far more than shouting, screaming or smacking. He would do anything he was asked as long as there was a treat clutched in my hand. He taught me that having a sense of humour was the best way of dealing with any sadness or worry. A dog has an uncanny ability of turning a lonely moment into one where there's a companion who never takes life too seriously for too long. Taffy had the trick, as Butch does now. A head cocked to the side, ears erect, eyes full of love and mischief – one could even say a cheeky grin. You can't stay miserable when faced with such innocent enthusiasm.

Taffy even managed to make me laugh during one of the greatest moments of shame and humiliation in a now rather long lifetime. I must have been 10 or 11 and, even though by now he was at least five years old, he hadn't grown out of his puppy habit of gobbling up anything he found on the floor, no matter how seemingly unappetising. We'd just left the house and were walking along the pavement on our way for a tour around the cemetery with Mum (I'd persuaded her it was an interesting place to visit) when he desperately needed the toilet.

The mystery of what had happened to the stocking my mother had said was missing from under her bed was revealed. The only way we managed to get the whole thing out was for me to step on it as it emerged and my mother to walk him away from me. Passers by looked on in open-mouthed astonishment as my mother and I giggled, red-faced, and tried to explain we were not indulging in a perverse form of doggy torture. Taffy looked round at me with a look of grateful and slightly shameful thanks. I was helpless with laughter.

I also found that even the most devoted and faithful companion needs a life of his own. It was probably genetic, given his father was something of a tramp, as, I suppose, was his mother, but there were times when he would nip out into the 'dogproof' garden and simply disappear. He'd be gone for several nights on the tiles, much to my dismay, but would always return ragged and exhausted, no doubt leaving many other little ginger mongrels dotted around the town.

I was in my second year at university when I came home for Christmas to be greeted as usual by his cheery, wagging welcome. Throughout our lives together he had always seemed to know when I was due and had never been absent from his place by the door where he waited for me. When I came home from school he was there, following me as I dropped my satchel in the hall, ran upstairs to change and took him for his walk. After a trip out in the evening, he appeared to hear me get off the bus a five-minute walk away and would leave his place by the fire to be ready for the opening door, and now, even though I spent long weeks away, he still seemed to anticipate my arrival.

On this occasion   I was 20, he was nearing 16 – he sat on my lap watching television all evening and nipped into the garden for his late night wee before bed. I didn't worry too much when he didn't come in. I guessed he'd gone off to a party some-where and would soon be back. I never saw him again. He hadn't been too well and my father reck-oned he was the kind of independent spirit who would have wanted to go off and die alone. I was inconsolable and vowed never to fall in love with a dog for a second time.

His death was the first bereavement I'd ever had to face and his sudden absence, so final, seemed unbearable. We had grown up together and shared so many adventures and so much quiet, cuddly pleasure. I couldn't imagine it would ever be possible to fill the gap he left, and to do so, despite advice from all around that the best way to deal with the death of a pet was to get another one, it felt that to try and replace him would be a betrayal of all the devotion he'd given.

For ten whole years I remained faithful to his memory. I finished university and managed to wheedle my way into the career I longed for. It was not easy in the early 1970s for a young woman to get herself on to the broadcasting ladder at the BBC. They turned me down once after a disastrous interview when my mugged-up knowledge of the technical side of the business far outshone my familiarity with the current events of the day. Lesson learned: never go to an interview without having devoured every available newspaper that morning. I eventually managed to persuade the manager at BBC Radio Bristol that I had potential and started at the very bottom of the ladder as a copy-taker in the newsroom.

Much as I loved radio, he persuaded me that survival in such a volatile industry meant having a wide range of journalistic skills – he taught me how to do radio, encouraged me to write and then packed me off to television in Southampton, which is why I found myself working as a reporter and presenter on the regional news programme, *South Today*. I'd met a dashing young naval officer, David Forgham, bought my own house on the edge of the New Forest and he was in the process of moving in (he's still here thirty years on) when the news editor announced he needed someone to cover the New Forest agricultural show. I drew the short straw. A dull day of watching farmers parade their prize cattle around the ring and plump little girls whipping their Thelwell ponies over the jumps.

I was perched on a shooting stick, bored and waiting for the cameraman to finish filming the 'idyllic' country scene. He was brilliant but laboriously slow so we called him, partly out of impatience and partly admiration, 'Every Frame's a Rembrandt'. I spotted a large, untidy woman, hair falling out of her carelessly pinned French pleat, striding purposefully across the field, heading for the dog show. Trotting elegantly by her side was the cutest thing I'd ever seen on four legs. It was small, grey, square-nosed, with floppy ears that flapped up and down as it ran and a short, docked tail that wagged incessantly. It bore a strong resemblance to the Tramp from *Lady and the Tramp* and I was intrigued. It was a breed I'd never seen before.

I chased after the woman and caught her, breathless, just before she got to the show ring. She explained that it was a miniature Schnauzer. She was in a hurry. She was due to show right now. Yes, she had a litter of pups. She lived in a caravan in a field in the lee of Salisbury Cathedral. I'd be welcome to go and have a look. She'd be easy to find.

I rushed home after work, brimming with excitement at the thought of bundling David into the car, driving to Salisbury and coming home with my new best friend in my lap. Happily for the continuation of our relationship, he expressed no objection whatever to the acquisition of a dog. I'm not sure we would have survived had he said he hated dogs and couldn't envisage coping with the responsibility. It would not have boded well for his future reliability as a hands-on father.

* * *

There are, in my experience, two types of dog breeder. There are those who do it not for the love, but the money. The bitches and pups are kept in cages and have little or no human contact. Then there are those who live in utterly disorganised and far less than hygienic chaos, but their animals – no matter how many they have – are part of the family. They're petted and cuddled and any small indiscretion in the toilet department is either ignored or dealt with swiftly and without fuss.

This breeder, Diana, was of the latter variety. They had owned a farm in the path of the as yet unbuilt M27 and had been compulsorily purchased in favour of the road. They had bought the land in Salisbury and were in the process of building their own house, brick by laborious brick. The caravan housed husband and wife, two strapping sons and several giant and numerous miniature Schnauzers. We were reluctant to take the proffered grubby seats and worried what we might catch from the cups of coffee which appeared immediately, but the puppies were bright, healthy, friendly and affectionate. The one I'd seen at the show appeared to recognise me.

He leaped on to my lap, licked me profusely and promptly fell asleep. He was perfect. His colour was grey, known in the trade as pepper and salt, and a boy, which was what I wanted.

Another, a more unusual black colour and a bitch, jumped on to David. There was some discussion about which we would take. I won. We paid £200 – a colossal sum in those days, which meant no dinners out and probably no holiday abroad that year – and drove home with William, who seemed to suffer no separation anxiety from his mother or his siblings. He was William from the moment we saw him, named after the character in the Richmal Crompton books we'd both loved as children. Our dog was 'Just William' from the word go – cheeky, naughty and irrepressibly amusing.

David was clearly delighted with him, but couldn't stop talking about 'the little black one' we'd rejected. The next morning we took William into the garden for his first lessons in house training – it was a Saturday, so we didn't have to worry about going to work – and David kept on going on about her.

'You know,' he finally came up with the clincher, 'it's all very well keeping a dog when you both have to go to work, but it's not really fair. It would be much better if we had two dogs and then they'd keep each other company when we were out.'

We rang Diana immediately, found another £200 we didn't really have and went off to Salisbury to collect her. She, it turned out, had already been named as Diana had half intended to keep her for breeding. She was known in the family as Hairy Mary. So, William and Mary. Names that went so well together. It seemed to bode well.

And so, for the next eighteen years, William and Mary were the best companions anyone could wish for. They took the arrival of two boisterous boys in their stride and were as playful and as gentle as any dog could be. William's only fault was a tendency to be the canine equivalent of Houdini, able to escape from any confinement and take himself on a date. I recommended castration, as advised by our vet. David would hear nothing of it. He had no objection to Mary being spayed to avoid any unwanted inbreeding, but the thought of emasculating William was beyond the pale.

Quite how he survived the move from Hamp-shire to Clapham is a mystery to me. We were super careful about keeping him in as we lived dangerously close to the South Circular. Nevertheless, there would frequently be phone calls from the other side of Clapham Common asking us to pick up our dog, usually after I'd opened the door a mere crack to pass a cheque out to the milkman or the paper boy and William had managed to squeeze through a gap that wouldn't have accommodated a mouse. We did, though, discover from a neighbour that he had a surprising degree of road sense. He was spotted trot-ting along our road to the zebra crossing, waiting on the pavement for a gap in the traffic and then scurry-ing hell for leather across the Common. He should never have lived for so long, but he did.

Just as I had grown up with Taffy, my two sons, Edward and Charlie, enjoyed the fun of the long walks a dog forces upon your daily routine and the comfort of a live and loving cuddly toy. The boys learned to care for an animal and treat it with respect, as I had. On Ed's first trip to the vet for annual booster jabs – he was two – he left the surgery announcing that was what he would do when he grew up – become a dog doctor. He's now 27 and a qualified vet.

The dogs were endlessly tolerant with the rough and tumble created by two small boys. Mary was patience personified – never minding when the ball sailed over her head to be caught by a giggling boy on the other side of the garden during a game of piggy in the middle with a dog as the piggy, chasing a football out on the Common like a mini Maradona and resigning herself to any tickling or ear tugging a toddler might choose to inflict. William's policy was to teach an over-enthusiastic tease a little lesson. He would growl and grab a flailing arm, crossly, in his mouth. The boy would squeal, I would rush to the child in fear of a bite and find not so much as the tiniest tooth mark in the delicate skin.

We were a family of six and the dogs went with us everywhere. We rarely went abroad for holidays as we hated leaving them, even with a house sitter. Our best vacation ever was a tour around the Dingle Peninsula in Ireland in a horse-drawn caravan. No space at all in the caravan, so boys and dogs were

deliriously happy at being able to share their beds –
William and Mary were usually confined to the
kitchen at night – and tons of space outdoors on
exquisite, long, isolated, empty, golden beaches. The
four of them would chase each other in and out of
the sea, barking and squealing with absolute delight
at the freedom they were able to enjoy.

It was Mary who began to deteriorate first. We
had moved to the Peak District when Ed was 11,
Charlie 7 and the dogs already in their teens. David
and I were two Northerners born and bred, drawn
home and wanting to give our sons the benefit of a
similar Northern Grammar School education to the
one to which we had access.

For William and Mary it meant a few traffic-free
years of nothing but garden and fields and the occasional run after a rabbit. Eventually, at the grand old
age of 18, Mary became so ill and incontinent, we
took her to the vet who said senility was simply shut-
ting everything down and it would be better to put
her out of her misery. We held her close whilst the
lethal injection was administered – the boys, bravely
trying to conceal how heartbroken they were by

sitting in the waiting room rather than watching the ghastly final act – and eventually David and I wrapped her in her blanket and we carried her lifeless body home and dug a grave at the bottom of the garden.

We laid her to rest with due ceremony. The four of us stood at her graveside, crying and laughing at happy memories of her skills as a footballer, insatiable appetite for anything sweet that might fall at her feet and love of rolling in anything unspeakably smelly she could find. William stood at my side, erect, like an old soldier, paying his own solemn and silent tribute.

William was a picture of utter misery without his lifelong companion. On the following Sunday night I had to leave home to travel to work in London, my weekly commute, knowing he might not be there when I got back. On the Wednesday, David called to say William's breathing was laboured. Should he take him to the vet? I begged him to hang on if at all possible until I got home the next day.

When I arrived my beloved little fella hauled himself out of his bed and dragged himself across the kitchen to greet me. It was obvious he was in some pain and distress. We wrapped him up in his bed and he sat on my knee in the car whilst David drove. The boys were at school. Now, if there was one thing William hated above all others, it was the vet. He detested his annual jabs and it was the only time he ever made a fuss about anything.

As we turned the corner into the road where the surgery is situated, he pulled himself up with great difficulty, licked my face and died in my arms. I have no doubt he knew where he was heading and was determined he was not going to depart this life igno-miniously with a needle stuck into his vein. We turned around and sobbed all the way home.

By the time we arrived and built up enough strength and courage to go down to the bottom of the garden and dig a grave alongside Mary's, it was dark and raining. Tears poured down our cheeks as, wet and bedraggled, we laid him down. A car passed, flashing its headlights on to us. We caught the look of alarm in the driver's face. We looked at each other. Only that week the crimes of Fred and Rose West had been uncovered, and here we were, digging a grave and burying a body at the dead of night. The situation was so macabre, we couldn't help laughing. From beginning to end, William had given us nothing but constant amusement. How we would miss him. We vowed there would be no more dogs. The sense of loss was too great.

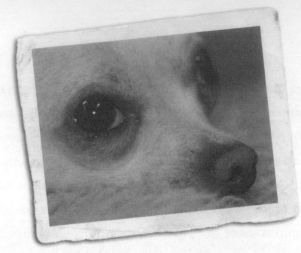

Chapter Two

Honey, I Want a Chihuahua

Time does heal the sadness, and those resolutions never to feel this bereft again fade and are almost forgotten in the chaos that is middle-aged life with a job to do, late teenagers to guide, nurture and ferry about and elderly parents to support and care for. I had hardly thought about getting another dog as every waking moment was filled with responsibility.

The boys were stuck in a house in a remote part of the countryside which had been perfect for adventurous youngsters, but less appealing when school friends were spread over a wide area of Cheshire and sleepovers and parties became an essential part of their social life. David and I became unpaid taxi drivers and sources of help and information on subjects as widespread as Shakespeare, Buddhism and quantum physics. Our brains were permanently in overdrive whilst, at the same time, dealing with the mundane everyday – shopping, cooking, making sure their shoes still fit.

As they reached 17 and passed their driving tests we looked forward to a little more free time. It was not to be. My parents became increasingly needy of support as my mother's Parkinson's worsened, and one day out of every weekend was taken up with the hour and a half drive to Barnsley and back to offer whatever care and cheer we could. By the time the end came for them and I had to face the loss of my parental rock – a gaping emotional hole that still, four years on, I find difficult to rationalise – I was forced to deal with my diagnosis of breast cancer.

People often ask me how I coped with it all, and the only answer is that you just do. Up to that point I had led something of a charmed life – lovely family, great job and the rudest of health, but always, in the back of my mind, there had been a sense that somehow, some day, this presumptuous little working-class lass from Barnsley would be caught out. Life had no right to be this good. I can't say I was surprised when all hell appeared to break loose at once. Both David and I were permanently over-whelmed and exhausted, falling into bed at night with barely a word exchanged between us and waking the next morning, dreading whatever new trial fate might dish out.

Slowly, but surely, the pressures eased. The grief was less acute as the months passed by. The children did well in their exams and were all but up and off to university, work and travel. The chemotherapy ended, my hair grew back thicker and bouncier than ever and the brilliant doctors who treated me declared my prognosis good. I felt well, and some of the old energy reasserted itself. The empty nest was not the disastrous cavern I had feared.

I began to get used to (and secretly rather enjoy) it, when that Titanic pile of shoes cluttering up the hallway came to an end; when the strains of drum and bass no longer emanated from the bedrooms; when there wasn't the constant need to be shrieking 'Turn that music down, will you'; and we could finally choose not to cook tonight's meal if we didn't really feel like it. But we were in no way fulfilling the promise we made to each other to take advantage of our lack of responsibilities and get out more – maybe even embark on some travel ourselves. We were becoming middle aged and more than a little staid.

Perhaps it was a necessary period of regrouping after the chaos of the hectic years that we had now tried to put behind us. There is a point in middle age when you realise you are not invincible. You've watched your parents deteriorate and are only too well aware that you will be next. Some days we sat opposite each other at the kitchen table and wondered whether, without the children and their future to discuss every day, we would ever again find anything to say to each other that wasn't depressing. What, we wondered, could replace the youth and energy they had brought to our lives? Of course, we were still occupied by phone calls, emails and the occasional visit, the requests for help and advice and sporadic donations from the bank of Mum and Dad, but it became increasingly apparent that an injection of something we were at a loss to define was necessary to re-invigorate us.

My thoughts, inevitably, turned towards canine companionship. Quite what put the idea of a Chihuahua into my head I'm not sure, as I've found myself strongly disapproving of the Chi celebrity culture that seems to have gripped Hollywood. I doubt there's ever been a dog that's enjoyed so much publicity since Lassie popularised the collie in *Lassie Come Home*.

The Taco Bell talking Chihuahua took America by storm, advertising Mexican Fast Food. Reese Witherspoon carried Bruiser – dressed in pink – in her designer handbags in *Legally Blonde*. In 2008 *Beverley Hills Chihuahua* was a hot success at the box office. Paris Hilton was rarely seen without Tinkerbell or Bambi. Madonna had Chiquita, Britney Spears sported Lucky and the movie hard man, Mickey Rourke, is said to own seven of the breed.

It's Rourke with whom I feel most sympathy. A reporter from the London *Times* described arriving at his small house in New York to be greeted by 'seven dogs, yipping, yapping and woofing and gleefully tripping over each other'. Rourke talks of the company his animals provide in what seems to have been a lonely and difficult life and his sense of responsibility even towards Jaws – a mean-spirited dog he took home from a rescue centre after it bit him on the lip. It had, he said, been ill treated by its previous owner. And he was clearly broken-hearted when his first dog, Loki, died at the age of 18 just before he was due to appear at the Oscar ceremony after his nomination as best actor.

Rourke says he chooses such small dogs because they tend to live longer and he becomes very attached. There is nothing of the designer doggie in its Gucci bag about him that's become such a feature of the Paris Hilton school of ownership that's had such a profound influence on the popularity of the breed.

The purchase of Chihuahuas in recent years has rocketed, despite the ever-escalating cost. You can expect to pay anything from £500 to £2,500, depending on the quality of the animal's pedigree – the average price seems to be around £1,000. But the British Chihuahua Club's Rescue Association reports more small dogs in need of rehoming than ever before. The internet small ads sites are full of notices for 'my cute little Chihuahua … 1 year old … genuine reason for sale'. In other words – 'Oops … this is a real dog. It's not a toy. It makes messes in the house and I couldn't be bothered to train it properly.' Small dogs are notoriously difficult to housetrain in the early days without constant supervision.

Alternatively you can read into the advert, 'Oops, it snapped at my two-year-old' … Chihuahuas are too small themselves to withstand the sometimes casual cruelty of a small child. Or, of course, it could simply be 'Oops, oh dear, he grew too big to fit in my handbag.' Britney is reported to have got rid of Lucky after he snapped at her then partner, Kevin.

Strangely, the more I read about the 'problem' Chihuahua the more intrigued I became. How could such a little animal be so fêted on the one hand and so demonised on the other? An article in the *Guardian* newspaper's G2 section headlined 'LA's

Chihuahua problem? Blame it on Paris' reported that Chihuahuas are now replacing pit bulls as the breed most often left at Californian shelters, with one San Francisco home telling the *LA Times* that, at current growth, the shelter will be 50 per cent Chihuahuas within months. 'Animal welfare workers are calling it the "Paris Hilton Syndrome" after the celebutante whose obsessive acquisition of handbag portable dogs has inexplicably encouraged their popularity among people who don't actually house the mutts in chandelier-hung scale models of their Beverley Hills mansions.'*

For me, living an oddly itinerant lifestyle that involves my weekly commute from the home in the Peak District I call Wuthering Heights to Wuthering Depths, the slightly grim, somewhat Bohemian basement flat in London, a small dog is essential for ease of transportation. Nor have I ever really been fond of big, powerful dogs, and Rottweilers and Alsatians really rather scare me. My son Ed the vet (I always feel slightly ashamed when I say that; it's like the old

* *Guardian*, 8 January 2010.

Jewish mother joke: she's in the swimming pool watching her boy and shouts, 'Help, help, my son, the doctor, is drowning!') goes by the old Barbara Woodhouse mantra – 'there are no bad dogs, only bad owners', but the only nasty experience I've ever had with a dog was during my childhood and the dog was an Alsatian.

Our local vicar, his wife and children lived in a huge, imposing Victorian vicarage, reminiscent of the scary house on the hill in Hitchcock's *Psycho*, and he began by owning one Alsatian as protection against intruders which eventually, as seems to happen with real dog lovers, became two, then four and eventually they were the proud owners of six of the breed – all brought up around their children and seemingly well trained and with the most gentle and accommodating temperaments.

I became involved with the family as a result of my loosely Church of England mother – she never went to church herself, but seemed to think it essential for my moral development. She insisted I go to Sunday school and be confirmed. I doubt she ever predicted I would be drawn to a short period of religious mania – I adored the drama of the High Church services and revelled in the bells, smells, music, intoned poetry of the services and the delicious cadences of the King James Version of the Bible – but she was patently delighted that I began to ally myself as a friend with the vicar's children rather than with the somewhat scruffy, 'common' (her word, not mine) oiks who raced around our street, spoke in broad Yorkshire accents and had little ambition apart from the kitchen or the pit.

The dogs would always be around the large garden as we played and were rarely averse to being dressed in old hats and cardigans or put into prams and pushed around. But one day, as we all appeared to be playing merrily, the two older males began their own scrap for no reason we could deduce. The girl in the family – Jane – my closest friend, a pretty child with translucent skin, turned-up nose and a much envied golden ponytail, decided the best policy was to intervene and separate the animals in case they hurt each other. The underdog immediately slunk away as she leapt between them, shouting, 'Stop it, stop it now!' The bigger and stronger of the two growled, jumped towards her, put its paws on her shoulders and tore into her lovely face.

It immediately seemed to realise it had made a terrible mistake, turned and ran away. The rest of us looked on in paralysed horror as Jane screamed in pain. Her parents ran out to see what had happened, bundled her into the car and drove off to the hospital. The plastic surgeons did their best, but there was always an angry scar at the side of Jane's face, and the dog was put down. It was a salutary lesson in animal behaviour – the two should have been left to get on with their scrap – and I'm not sure I would ever entirely trust a dog with the size and power to create such havoc. Even now I shiver slightly if I see one approaching in the park.

Soon after, I stopped going there – I found it hard to cope with Jane's misery at the damage to her face and never again felt quite comfortable with the remaining animals. Eventually, they left the area and I lost touch with them completely.

So, a small dog it had to be. Friends with whom I shared my longing met my wittering about a really little dog being just the ticket with universal astonishment. They even went so far as to say they didn't see me as someone who would be so shallow as to mince about with a designer dog or ally myself with what they saw as nothing more than a yappy, irritating rat on a string.

Nevertheless I found myself drawn irresistibly to the 'Chihuahuas for Sale' personal ads every time I sat down at the computer and read everything I could lay my hands on about the nature of the breed. The more I read, the more convinced I became that this was the perfect companion for someone in middle age who was not as fit as she once had been. Easy to manage physically, maniacally devoted to their owner, too small to be around very little children, not too expensive to feed, generally enjoying robust health and happy to go on a long walk if that took your fancy or a slow stroll around the sitting room if you didn't feel up to a morning of violent exercise.

There was only one problem. David was absolutely adamant that he did not want another dog. During our first few years together, when the Royal Navy owned his time and could send him on a tour of duty at a moment's notice, it was I who took on the responsibility of looking after William and Mary and arranging childcare for Ed when he was a baby. It was David's longing to be a hands-on father who didn't have to be away for months on end that drove him to leave the service and, eventually, when trustworthy and affordable childcare became increasingly difficult to find, he decided to take on the children whilst I became the breadwinner. He'd had years where full-time care was his job. He now relished the freedom to go out if he wanted to without worrying about anyone else's needs. And that obviously meant, no dog.

In our relationship of thirty years' standing there has rarely been a major disagreement. We concurred on where to live, what kind of house we wanted, how to educate and discipline the boys, but this was becoming a serious problem. I didn't want to bring a living creature into the house if he would not be able to welcome it, but I was almost tempted to think I'd prefer the dog to him! Dogs don't do grumpy!

There's a theory, set out in *The Female Brain* by an American psychologist, Louann Brizendine, that

a post-menopausal woman loses her nurturing gene.
She's said to become selfish in a way she has never
been before and no longer feels it necessary to shop,
cook, clean and care for those around her. Her children are generally up and off and her husband or
partner can stand on his own two feet.

I can testify that it is to some extent true in rela-
tion to children and partners. I did get to a point
where I was only prepared to cook and wash clothes
or dishes strictly on a rota basis, but somewhere, deep
in my soul, was the need to have someone or something small, helpless and needy to look after.

And I was not alone. We went out to dinner one
evening with Gaynor and Ernie, friends of our age
who don't have children together. It's their second
marriage and Ernie's boys are grown up; Gaynor
hasn't had a child of her own. The conversation came
round to filling one's time as one approached late
middle age. The guys were all for working less hard,
finding their way around the golf course, being free,
at the drop of a hat, to see the world. Gaynor and I
could talk of nothing but a dog and possible arrangements for reliable and affordable dog care, should the

need arise. The nurture gene was only too present in both of us. Unsurprising, I guess, as psychologists describe the need to nurture as an essential part of the human condition, giving the lie to what was obviously nonsense about the gene diminishing as a woman gets older. I felt it as keenly in my mid fifties as I had heard the ticking of my biological clock in my early thirties.

I begged for a puppy for Christmas. I know, I'm not so stupid as to think a puppy should ever be bought for Christmas – it's after the festivities that so many end up in shelters, unwanted and unloved, when a family that has bought in haste begins to realise how much of a commitment a dog is. But I really thought they would see how much I seemed to need a dog and would give in and surprise me.

They seemed to find it amusing to watch me unwrap a robot puppy which walked around the floor, barked, whined, sat on command and was about as cuddly and comforting as a lump of cold steel. I didn't let them see me shed tears of disappointment. I did that in my bedroom, alone, and when the children were gone, after the holiday, I threw the stupid toy in the bin. And the house sank back into that cold, life-less emptiness I found so dispiriting.

All alone, I read about dogs and was delighted to spend an hour with a marvellous *Horizon* programme on BBC television called 'The Secret Life of Dogs'. It began to explain some of the reasons why I might be feeling so bereft and so full of longing. Research-ers have found that we respond to the face of a dog in much the same warm way as we respond to small babies. Experiments placed human beings into a brain scanner and found that the same area of the brain lights up when shown a picture of a human baby as is illuminated when a dog's face is shown. It doesn't happen if the picture is of an adult human. And indeed there are noteworthy similarities in the faces of babies and dogs – a high forehead, sweet little button nose and big, innocent eyes.

Most remarkably, researchers trying to under-stand why the dog has become man's (or woman's) best friend have learned how the dog was domesti-cated by conducting experiments with wolves and, separately, with silver foxes. First they tried to raise wolf cubs in a domestic environment in exactly the same way as tiny puppies. The wolves showed absolutely no inclination to behave in an acceptable manner. If the fridge door opened they simply dived in and took whatever they wanted, regardless of being told 'No'. They remained wild and independent. As one of the researchers who had cuddled, slept with and nurtured a wolf cub said rather ruefully as hers jumped up and took her meal from the table, tearing down the tablecloth and everything on it in the process, 'He just doesn't care.' Eventually the wolves in the experiment were returned to the sanctuary to be with their own kind as it was thought to be too dangerous to keep them at home. Conclusion? They couldn't be domesticated without a careful breeding programme.

My son Ed had close experience of this phenomenon when, during his year between school and university, he spent time at a wolf sanctuary in the mountains of Colorado. It was set up to rescue wolves who had mistakenly been bought as pets and had created havoc as they became fully grown. The most alarming animals he came across – indeed the only ones he felt presented any real danger to the people who cared for them – were the ones where, foolishly, an Alsatian had been crossed with a wolf. A wolf, he says, will never attack a human being unless it feels threatened. It will simply slink off in fear and seek its prey among sheep or cattle. A wolf dog is dangerous. It has the wolf's wild nature and the dog's total lack of fear of the human being.

Yet all dogs, I learned from the programme, owe their genetic inheritance to the wolf. The process of domestication has been researched in Russia at a university in Siberia in Novosibirsk. There, over a 50-year period, silver foxes, a naturally wild and potentially aggressive animal, have been bred based on their temperament. Only the least aggressive have been allowed to breed and, during the 50 years, the researchers have found each new generation becoming progressively more tame and changing their physical characteristics. Sometimes the colour has altered. In some cases the tail has become curly. They are, it seems, becoming dogs, and the conclusion is that a similar selective process was used to change the appearance and the temperament of the wolf.

The most incredible experiments involved a complex bit of recording equipment which shows the scientists which way we look at faces. For some reason we humans don't look straight at each other. We always look to our left when gazing at another person's face, which means we're looking at the right side of our subject. It apparently makes us easier to read. And, amazingly, the dog is the only animal to do exactly the same thing. It so wants to please us it has learned how to read our facial expression, our tone of voice, our vocabulary (most dogs at least know 'sit', 'bed', 'ball', 'fetch' or 'walkies') and one dog in the programme understood 300 words. Again, uniquely among animals, the dog can even follow our gestures, something not even our closest relative, the chimpanzee, can do.

When a chimp was offered treats hidden under cups it ignored the researcher's finger pointing towards the one that contained the morsel of food and simply went its own way. Dogs, even the youngest eight-week-old puppies, followed the finger and succeeded every time.

It's also been found that close physical contact with a dog produces the hormone oxytocin in both the owner and the dog. It's the same hormone that's produced when a woman gives birth and breastfeeds her baby. The French obstetrician, Michel Odent, calls it 'the love hormone'. It's been found to produce feelings of contentment and relaxation.

It doesn't surprise me to discover that people who have a close and affectionate relationship with a dog suffer less stress, are less likely to suffer a heart attack and, if they do, are more likely to recover. I'm not sure whether that's a result of the calming effect of the oxytocin and the frequent cuddles you get with a creature that offers and receives unconditional love or whether it's the fact that dog owners get out more because they have to be involved in more physical exercise than the non-dog owner who doesn't have to do 'walkies' three times a day, but the evidence is compelling. And it must be noted that during my years of dog ownership I never ailed a thing.

So, my arguments in favour of having another dog were bolstered by the science. There were other slightly alarming nuggets of information in the programme which I thought it might be profitable not to share with the partner I call, in less affection-ate moments, 'him indoors'. There are 8 million dogs in the UK alone, which is an awful lot of unwanted waste matter on pavements and in parks.

I have always held to being a responsible owner and never leave anything behind, remembering ghastly times when the children were young and we lived in London near Clapham Common. They would run, somersault, play football and cycle and inevitably bring home something unpleasant on their shoes or trousers. Horrid. The other truly scary statistic informs me the average dog owner invests £20,000 in their animal over its lifetime. That's the initial cost of the dog, insurance, vets bills, food, toys, beds and other paraphernalia. It's an amount I shall choose to ignore.

But all the stuff about the health-giving properties of dog ownership – now that was really useful. David had been the most attentive of carers during my nasty brush with those unwanted cancer cells. He stood by me manfully through discussions with the surgeon that no man should ever have to witness – a cold and matter-of-fact analysis of how best to remove a part of his partner's body of which both he and she are particularly fond. He was at my bedside when I was taken to theatre and still there when my morphine-addled brain began to come round and talk nonsense.

He brought me home and tucked me up. He was there for the chemotherapy sessions and held the bucket by my bed when the nausea kicked in. He had, I knew, had quite enough of caring and would do anything to make me take better care of myself than had been my habit in the past.

I needed to develop a strategy. It involved appearing rather depressed and down in the mouth. It was not, after all I'd been through, entirely a performance, although I confess now to playing it up a bit. I became reluctant to go out much. I developed a passion for a lie-in in the morning, a bit of a nap in the afternoon and then an early night. He was clearly worried that I was not as well in the hours spent at home as I appeared to be when I was trotting off to London to go to work, or seemed when he heard me coming out of the radio. I was obviously, I think he realised, short of something to occupy my time.

Eventually, he asked me what he could do to help me feel better. Bingo! I shamelessly played the cancer card. I told him I hoped to live for many more years – an aspiration he seemed to share. Fifteen to twenty, at least. I discussed my oncologist's assurance that, after the type of breast cancer I'd had and the subsequent treatment, my prognosis seemed to be good. A dog, with luck and good husbandry, would share most of those fifteen to twenty years, especially a Chihuahua, known for their longevity. A bright little dog would give me a reason to get up in the morning. It would force me to go out for walks and get the exercise I so desperately needed.

I would take it with me to keep me company in London. I would take full responsibility for everything that was necessary. I would sort out the vet and the injections (as David pointed out, that wouldn't be too much of a hardship as we had a vet living just around the corner and who, being our son, would be unlikely to charge us). I would do all the puppy training, cleaning up any accidents immediately. I would go and buy all the necessary equipment and do the weekly food shop. I would never expect him to do the walks unless he really wanted to. I would find someone responsible who would be pleased to take the dog in if we needed/wanted to go away on holiday ... health care ... everything. And most importantly it would cheer us up with a deliriously happy welcome every time we came home. He knew he'd been had.

Finally, after months of agonising, David said, 'Yes.'

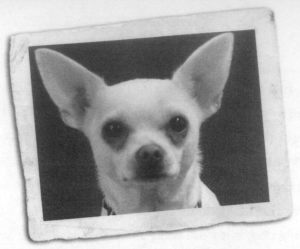

Chapter Three

That Doggie in the World Wide Window

I had become a virtual prisoner in my room, chained to the computer, scanning the one website I know is considered respectable with adverts for dogs for sale, Pets4Homes. Every day I clicked on: Type of animal? Dog. Breed? Chihuahua. Area? Manchester, Cheshire, Staffordshire … anywhere in this hungry search for the friend I hoped would be my close companion for the rest of my life.

I didn't care about colour, but I wanted a boy. I used to long for a daughter, but after raising two sons I'd got used to the testosterone around the house and what I can only describe as the straightforwardness of the male. Taffy was a guy, William was always my favourite of William and Mary. I wanted a little, loving dog, but I did want a lad!

He didn't have to be advertised as teacup size. I'm not sure I approve of breeding dogs that are impossibly small – destined to be carried in the handbag. He had to be home bred. I won't tolerate a puppy farm or any breeder that seems to be advertising lots of puppies where the bitches and their babies have been kept in cages. I also zoomed past the photos of dogs that were lying on red velvet cushions, had a TV remote by their side to indicate the smallness of their size or were dressed in outrageous little outfits.

I wanted a small-scale, sensible amateur breeder, one that advertised one litter of pups and assured the enquirer that the puppies were well socialised, having had lots of contact with family, and the parents could be seen. Kennel Club Registration is completely unnecessary for a pet who won't be shown or used for breeding. The puppy would have to have been vet checked and have had its first set of jabs, and it wouldn't be allowed to leave its mother until at least 12 weeks old.

And then, one cold morning in December 2007, three years ago now, I saw him. It was a litter of four puppies. There was a picture of each one. He was short-haired and all white, with enormous black eyes. His ears flopped down, his head was slightly to the side and his expression was quizzical, intelligent and, somehow, honest.

I called immediately. Yes, the white boy was still available. He was six weeks old, so wouldn't be available until mid-January. Yes, both parents belonged to the owner and could be seen. We could go round right away. I hustled David into the car and we drove to a housing estate in Wythenshawe, just south of Manchester. It's a name that generally makes me shudder. It's the site of the hospital where I go every year for my check-ups to make sure the cancer hasn't gone walkabout. If this worked out, it would be a relief to be able to associate it with pleasure rather than pain.

The owner of the pups, Gemma, answered the door immediately. She welcomed us warmly, invited us to sit down and motioned to the child's playpen in the corner of the room. Would we like to see the puppies? She kept them in the playpen to stop them chasing around all day and to give their mother some relief from their constant hassling. She lifted them out one by one and put them on the rug in front of us.

I knew him immediately and he scurried over to me and tried to scramble up my trousers. I picked him up. He fitted neatly into my hand. I held him close to my face and he licked my cheek. I was sunk and, curiously, I thought, so was he. It was what the French would call a *'coup de foudre'* – a lightning strike – it was mutual love at first sight.

I sensed rather more than mere acceptance in David. He was visibly melting. We asked to see the parents, and Gemma, who was quiet, pregnant and gentle, left the room to bring them in. First the father – hefty for a Chihuahua, with long, golden hair, intelligent eyes, an impressively bushy tail and a winning personality – raced into the room and greeted us amicably. A good omen.

Then the mother. She had short dark brown hair, was handsome, healthy and decidedly cross. She didn't want to be fondled and she certainly didn't want to be around the pups. I put her ill temper down to maternal exhaustion as they scurried around her begging for nourishment. I recall only too well how painful it can be to try and feed an offspring that has teeth, and she had four of them going at her all at once. I knew I had been hooked on the little one who'd chosen me before I'd even had a chance to review the parents. They simply confirmed that I hadn't been mistaken.

And David just looked on adoringly and asked to give the baby a cuddle. He snuggled into David's hand, looking even tinier and more vulnerable than he had in mine. How on earth was I going to manage to wait another six weeks before I took him home?

We agreed a price (don't ask!) and a date for collection and Gemma asked what we might call him. 'Butch,' said David half-jokingly, as the name seemed so incongruous given his tiny frame, but it stuck. I think I may have acceded partly out of gratitude that David had given in to my longing for a dog, partly to give him some sense of ownership and partly to demonstrate that I had retained some of the sense of humour that had been missing somewhat in the previous few miserable years. There wasn't a great deal to make either of us laugh or smile as we struggled with my life-threatening illness and watched our sons take much of the life and soul of our little family party with them as they, quite rightly, made their own way in the world. I could see, even at that early stage, that Butch would bring back to us something of what had drained away.

Reluctantly we said goodbye, arranging a date in January to pick Butch up, and for the first of many times to come I saw a hint of sadness in Butch's face. You may think this is madness on my part, but whilst he can look dementedly happy and cheerful, he also has a morose look about him at times, generally mirroring my mood. I knew he was sorry to see us go. And sure enough, before he even joined us, David and I had something to talk about other than cancer treatments, repairs to the house and who does the washing up. Just as our conversation was once full of cheery chatter about our sons, we now had someone else to make plans for. And now we could look forward, rather than looking back nostalgically to the past.

The days were full of preparations for Christmas – no fear of any robot dogs appearing this time. The children came home for the celebrations, so the house was full of cheer and energy again, if only temporarily. Friends came to stay for New Year and it was over breakfast in the kitchen on New Year's Day, when I stood up from the table to make more coffee, that pain ripped through my left thigh. It felt as though someone had stuck a hot knife deep into the muscle and I cried out, thinking I must have stood awkwardly and pulled something. I hobbled about for the rest of the morning, staying in the car whilst the others walked around the grounds of Chatsworth House and even shortening the visit to the Chatsworth Farm Shop, usually one of the most pleasurable things to do on a lazy day off.

We bought venison, home-bred lamb, sausages and fancy preserves – all wildly overpriced, but with an ersatz aristocratic air about them. Then to Bakewell for a cup of coffee and a cake. It's always a favourite when friends come up from London. I've shown off my knowledge of the history of Chatsworth and the marvellous Elizabethan Derbyshire businesswoman, Bess of Hardwick, whose best beloved house it was. Four husbands, and she managed to marry up significantly each time.

We'd had the usual cheap and silly jokes about Bakewell tarts and I'd managed a rather tired giggle, but my progress through the little town, busy with end-of-season shoppers and still bedecked in Christmas lights and colours, was painfully slow. I couldn't wait to get home and persuade the assembled company of the delights of a nice sit down in front of low-brow TV. I could feel my New Year's resolution to get fit and thin already slipping through my fingers.

Everyone tried to reassure me that it would just be a strained muscle, but in bed, alone that night, I felt the anxiety rising. A sudden, unexpected and inexplicable pain to anyone who's had cancer can only mean one thing. The nasty little cells have gone walkabout. They must have gone to my bones. All my plans to look ahead with Butch and take him with me on my trips to London where we would have long walks in Regent's Park to complement our trekking across the hills of home seemed to be slipping away uncontrollably. How could I take on the responsibility of a dog if I was going to die?

And so the nights went, full of fears I didn't dare name to anyone else. In the daytime I carried on moving about with a slight limp, finding getting in and out of cars brought searing pain and making the long trek up the slope from the platform to the concourse at Euston Station feel like climbing Everest. It's strange that I would say to anyone else going through such anxiety, 'Go to the doctor, get it checked out,' but, somehow, when it's yourself and you've already been through a year of debilitating treatment, the ostrich approach seems more appealing. I just grinned and bore it, accusing myself of hypochondria.

On 12 January 2008 my diary records '<u>PICK UP BUTCH</u>' in huge, underlined, capital letters. I had somehow convinced myself that the pain would turn out to be nothing serious and that I would be able to manage what was, after all, a very small dog. I'd spent the intervening week or so reading everything I could about settling in a new puppy – it was such a long time since I'd done it – and had bought him a cosy bed, loads of cuddly toys, his own dishes, lots of Tesco's finest for puppies and a box designed for a cat with a sheepskin rug for him to lie on as I transported him home.

I rang Gemma's doorbell, only having struggled slightly to get out of the car, and heard excited yapping inside. He had grown enormously – pretty much doubled in size – but would still sit quite comfortably in my hand. Despite the increase in size, his ears continued to flop over – the book said they wouldn't stand up till five or six months old – and he was really quite round, almost chubby. As he ran around excitedly he fell over his feet, rolled and bounced like a little animate ball. He was adorable. Again there was that sign of recognition, a tacit agreement between us that we were meant for each other and he had been waiting for me to fetch him. I swept him up from the floor, my heart swelling with delight at holding him close, and the pain forgotten.

One of his siblings had gone already. His mother looked really rather relieved to be seeing the back end of her litter. She appeared much less grumpy than last time I saw her. I popped Butch into his container, hating having to bundle him away, but knowing driving would be safer that way, shut the door on him, said goodbye to Gemma and carried him with infinite delicacy towards the car, opening the door on the passenger side, lowering him tenderly on to the seat and fixing the seatbelt around the box. I didn't remember feeling this anxious when I took my first baby home from hospital. He just seemed so tiny and so vulnerable.

During the long ride home my concentration as a driver left a great deal to be desired. Butch cried pitifully, already missing his family and wondering why, for the first time ever, he was locked up in a strange environment with neither human nor animal warmth to cuddle up to. I was tempted to take him out and have him curl up on my lap, but he wasn't used to travelling in a car and I worried that he would be a dangerous distraction and we'd end up in a ditch somewhere.

The advice in the book was to use the box, even at home, as a sanctuary for the dog. I set out with the very best of intentions. When we got home David was there to welcome us. He'd sneakily been off to Pets Are Us and bought more toys – a long, white, sausage-shaped, furry sheep and a squeaky rubber pig, to which Butch took an immediate shine.

In fact he immediately seemed to recognise the kitchen as home and marched around sniffing at this and that, confronting our two cats, Snooker and Black Cat (the kids wanted to call him Julio after some American skateboarder, a name I hated, so he remained Black Cat or just Kit), backing away as they established that they were top of the pecking order, so he'd better watch himself, and then sitting at my feet whimpering until I took him on to my lap where he promptly fell asleep. He refused to be moved except, seemingly still asleep, to wriggle himself under my sweater.

It felt so good to have a little, warm creature snuggled so close again. There really is nothing like a dog for comforting reassurance. It was immediately clear that my habit of wearing black would have to change. White, shorthaired dogs and black clothes are no mix. I'd have to rifle through the wardrobe for more colourful garb that wouldn't show his hairs. My surgical oncologist told me he always knew when his patients were getting better when they wore lipstick, got their hair done and abandoned black. Butch was already setting me back on the road of cheeriness.

Toilet training with any new animal is always a priority, and the book was not encouraging when it came to Chihuahuas. Very small dogs are, apparently, pretty hard to train. They find it difficult to hang on for as long as a bigger animal. They won't soil their own bed, nor will they make a mess directly in front of you, but even when they've cottoned on to the fact that you don't do it in the middle of the rug, they may slope off into the corner of the room as they think they've gone a long way to find a private spot. Even the average sitting room feels like crossing the Sahara to such a small creature. The advice is to take the puppy out to the same spot in the garden every hour or so, praise them lavishly each time they perform and make them spend the night in the cage, working on the principle that their own bed is sacrosanct.

Butch did his very best to comply with my demands about cleanliness, but he hated having to go outside. Oh, why did I have to find him in December, and why do we have to live in the North West where rain is such a regular feature of the weather? He is not a dog for the great outdoors and he finds getting wet and cold a most unattractive prospect. Nevertheless, we stuck to our programme and every hour we popped out and he seemed to be getting the message. He certainly enjoyed the vigorous pats and joyous 'Good boys!' that I showered upon him each time he performed.

He had to be fed small amounts every three hours – Chihuahuas have a tendency to suffer from hypoglycaemia or low blood sugar if they're not topped up regularly, and he expended so much energy, bounding around, I needed to keep him full. Couldn't have him passing out. Even when a Chihuahua is an adult, you can't get away with just one meal a day, which is generally the case with most dogs. It was immediately clear why he had become so roly poly. He loved his food, waited in shivering excitement, standing on my feet as I dished up, looking up most winningly and hungrily and gobbling down every morsel in record time. Out we went, poo and wee wee, and back indoors as fast as his little wet legs could carry him. Sit down, jump on to my lap, fall asleep. By ten o'clock I was completely exhausted, and it was only Day One of our training programme. I announced I was off to bed.

'So, what are you going to do with Butch?' asked David, almost certainly knowing that the answer will not be, 'I'm going to leave him in the kitchen.' We've had our own rooms since the children were small. Charlie, number two son, developed an irritating habit of launching himself from his cot, crawling along the corridor and climbing into our bed before he was a year old. He would tuck down between us and scratch David's back with his toenails, making his claim on my undivided attention. Eventually it became too much for David.

It was a bit of a difficult conversation when he hesitantly proffered, 'Would you mind very much if I moved into the spare room?' Initially I minded very much. My parents had never spent a night apart during their entire marriage, except when Dad had to travel for work, and, as theirs seemed the ultimate in happy and contented unions, my partner not wanting to share my bed seemed to be the first step towards disaster.

It was only when I began to realise that I could read to my heart's content without hearing a grumbling, 'I can hear you turning the pages', could have the radio on or off at will and would not be woken up in the middle of the night by his snoring or his pinching my nose because of mine that I began to appreciate 'a room of one's own'. I'm now pretty certain that one of the reasons we've lasted so long is because we both get a decent night's sleep and I, ever the self-centred only child, have my own space with my own things and the luxury of being able to spread myself out without fear of becoming entangled in someone else or dragging off the duvet. It's my room, I can do exactly as I please.

And that, of course, includes my own dog! So on that first important night we went to the garden at the last minute, I tucked him into his catbox with one of his cuddly toys and set him down at the side of my bed, wishing him a good night and turning off the light. The whimpering began almost immediately and I knew I should just ignore it – that eventually he would tire and fall asleep till morning. But he seemed so wee and cried so pathetically. I opened the door to the cage and lifted him out. Immediately he pushed his nose under the duvet and with all his strength, looking like a mole burrowing under the lawn, up, down, up, down, he tucked himself in until he was finally satisfied he was cosy, warm and safe, and fell asleep. From that night on he's been my hot water bottle.

Six a.m. and he was licking my nose, jiggling about, saying, 'Come on, hurry up, it's time we got going.' And I, who have always followed the Somerset Maugham dictum – 'One should always do two things each day that one hates – going to bed and getting up' – found myself leaping out of bed with an entirely unfamiliar joy and enthusiasm.

The pain in the leg persisted, at its worst first thing in the morning, and we were a little slow getting down the stairs, but I carried him, not sure he was yet capable of doing stairs on his own, took him outside, fed him breakfast and tucked him into my arms again to go up and have my shower. He sat on the rug by the side of the shower and watched in bemused astonishment as I chose to stand under a torrent of water. He evidently thought his new mistress was quite mad and peed on the rug in protest. I did as instructed by the book and ignored his mistake, wrapping myself in a towel to pop him outdoors and wiping up and disinfecting the mess with no comment. It seemed we had a bit of a distance to go before the message would finally sink in.

The leg was not getting any better and my plan to take Butch with me on my weekly trips to London had to be abandoned. I could barely take responsibility for myself, let alone for the two of us. A friend had recommended a stick might help until it got better, so I had bags and the rather elegant, floral cane I bought to carry. No way could I manage Butch, inexperienced traveller as he was. Neither he nor David seemed too unhappy about being left together, and Butch's effusive greeting when I finally came home from my two or three work days in the capital almost made up for how much I missed him whilst I was away.

He learned about snow, treading disdainfully through a substantial covering and rushing in at the earliest possible opportunity, again making no bones about his distaste for any outdoor excursion that involved getting cold or wet. David came back from the shops with a woollen coat with a fur collar – the smallest size available – and even then it swamped his diminutive frame. Suddenly Dave was being softer than I would have been. In my canine world dogs are dogs and were given fur to keep them warm – they don't wear coats. Butch seemed to agree, wriggling about in a supreme effort to get the thing off. This was not difficult as it hung on him so loosely, but then he'd shiver ostentatiously whenever he went out and couldn't wait to get back to his favourite spot, apart from my lap, lying by the Aga alongside Black Cat, who seemed to have accepted that Butch was to be a permanent fixture, stopped spitting at him and threatening to scratch his eyes out and learned how to tease him mercilessly. David filmed them playing in the garden.

The cat would hide in the bushes as Butch ran around on a fine day, enjoying expending his phenomenal energy. The cat would let his tail hang out and waggle it around. Butch would make to leap at it, at which point the cat, cartoon-like, would whip around, all four paws akimbo and in the air, and scare Butch out of his wits. Even in the cold we would sit in garden chairs, wasting endless hours of time watching the show.

Eventually I could ignore the pain no longer and made an appointment on 21 January to see my GP. She is a woman I've trusted for more than 15 years and she is particularly sympathetic to concerns about cancer. She's had it herself – twice. She examined my thigh and wiggled it about, muttering endless reassurance about her certainty that we were absolutely not dealing with secondaries in the bone.

She seemed pretty convinced that I had, unknowingly, done myself an injury. She arranged for me to have an X-ray of the femur, the big bone in the thigh. There was a risk that my bone density may not be what it was after the abandonment of HRT at the cancer diagnosis and the requirement that I now take a tablet each day which would reduce the amount of oestrogen in my body. The anti-oestrogen medication was designed to protect me from any further tumour developing in the other breast, but it might possibly make the bones brittle. Perhaps, I thought, if the bone was weak, I may have cracked it, which would account for the pain.

Huge relief when the results came back negative for bone cancer, so the discomfort, which was getting worse all the time, must be muscular. I became increasingly irritated with the impact of the pain on my mobility. I found it harder and harder to get about easily, so the doctor recommended I try physiotherapy and referred me to Ruthie.

Ruthie has blonde, cropped hair, is awesomely fit and extremely beautiful. She has moved to our part of the world from the Midlands to be with her boyfriend, but has so far spent most of her career as the physio at Leicester Tigers – one of Britain's premier rugby clubs. I can only imagine what a stir this blonde bombshell must have caused among the crowds when she ran on to the pitch with her bandages and embrocation when one of the big boys needed treatment.

For several weeks, twice each week, I duly attended her sessions and she massaged and manipulated, giving me exercises which I tried to perform religiously, but which generally reduced me to a jelly-like, tearful heap. And things didn't get better. They got worse. Much worse. The pain that began in the left leg now seemed to have spread into the right. I considered abandoning the pretty stick and moving on to crutches. Far from regaining energy and the motivation to get out and about with Butch now the cancer seemed to be at bay, I felt like a doddery old lady, way beyond my years, huddled and hobbling, as I struggled to keep life as normal as possible. I was reluctant to take more time off work after all the absences of the previous year for surgery and chemotherapy. The BBC had been as supportive as an employer could be, although I wasn't sure how kindly they would take to more sick leave. I kept up the travelling to and from London, hauling myself on and off the trains, staggering from the train to the taxi at the station, waiting until the rushing crowds had passed whilst I made my slow progress and learning to get in and out of cars bum first as I could barely lift either leg to step in daintily.

David was getting more and more alarmed. He'd already spent nearly a year taking care of me during the treatment for cancer and now he saw me barely able to climb or descend the stairs at home. I crawled up on my hands and knees, weeping with anger, pain and frustration. I hadn't the energy to walk around the supermarket, so he was doing all the shopping again. I couldn't bear to stand long enough to cook a meal. The only light in my life was one bouncy, lively, loving little dog who snuggled into my lap and kissed my cheek with that slightly morose and mournful look that said, 'I know what you're going through, but don't worry. I don't mind.'

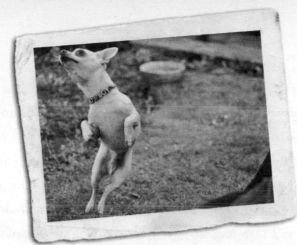

Chapter Four

Walkies?

It's generally expected that when a human being says 'Walkies!' to a dog in a voice that's light with enthusiasm and excitement, said dog will run around in the demented fashion frequently compared with a headless chicken. Butch, to my great immobile relief, was somewhat more circumspect. He opened one eye, stretched his limbs exaggeratedly, edged gingerly towards the door, checked the weather conditions and, even if there was no snow and it wasn't raining, but there was a distinct chill in the air, gave me a look that said, 'Naah! I'll just nip out quick, no need to come, and then when I'm done, gives us a cuddle.'

Every day the bond grew stronger and he followed my lead when it came to mood and mobility. As I crawled, slowly, up and down the stairs, he too took each step with studied care, even though I knew now, as he'd grown a little bigger, he could cover them in a leaping trice. He seemed to be aware that a wrong step on his part, getting under my feet, could send me tumbling with disastrous consequences. He went behind me, never wanting to alarm me or trip me up.

He was proving quick to learn and eager to please in every way, apart, that is, from lead training. He had no objection to his collar. It's a rather smart one, sent in by a listener to *Woman's Hour* who had read about him in my weekly newsletter. It's made of black leather and has the words 'Bad Boy' and a little crown attached in diamante. I vowed I would never put him in diamante, but it had such a strangely comic S&M air to it and looked so funny on this innocent, white little chap, I'm afraid it stuck. He seemed to rather like the joke.

Lead training was a disaster. I'd bought a light-weight expandable leash which I attached to the collar and carried him down the drive. The book had recommended taking a youngster a few yards from the gate, putting him down and encouraging him to follow you home. Butch was having none of it. Who would have thought something so small could have such strength of will? He dug his paws firmly into the ground and refused to budge. I tugged at the lead, saying, 'Come on, Butch.' He spun on the spot – round and round like a demented whirling Dervish. He looked so unhappy, I gave up, knowing it was going to be a while before we could go for proper walks in parks or on pavements and for now he was totally secure in the garden and the fields around us. I was going soft.

His exercise consisted of chasing a ball across the kitchen if the weather was poor or the garden if it was fine, whilst I sat and did nothing but throw the ball. He picked up a wide vocabulary – 'fetch', 'ball', 'bunny', 'pig', 'lamb', 'sit', 'wait' and 'bed'. He greeted every command with enthusiasm, went to fetch whatever he'd been asked for entirely appropriately, but his favourite word was 'bed'.

And he never headed towards the cosy little dog bed that was bought specially for him, but marched off towards the stairs and waited for me to join him. He followed me through my routine, bathroom, bedroom, bed, waiting patiently as I brushed my teeth and hair and undressed. Then, oh joy, he leapt on to my bed – quite a phenomenal height for one so wee – and snuggled down beside me under the duvet. He didn't seem to mind what time of day it was – there were days when I was so exhausted by the struggles with the pain I simply collapsed in the early afternoon. As long as he was by my side he was happy. The family found it disgusting and arguably unhealthy. I couldn't have cared less. He was my comfort – warm, living, breathing – and I was becoming every bit as devoted to him as he was to me.

I came across a poem by Rudyard Kipling which seemed perfectly tuned to the way I felt. To any sane person it seems hopelessly sentimental. To anyone who's ever made a close relationship with a dog it is an absolute truth. It will, I hope, be at least 16 years before we are to be parted, assuming that he, not I, will be the first to depart, but the poem made me think of how easily I'd fallen back in love again, despite being so torn apart when Taffy, William and Mary shuffled off this mortal coil. The poem goes:

> When the fourteen years which nature permits
> Are closing in asthma or tumour or fits
> And the vet's unspoken prescription runs
> To lethal chambers or loaded guns,
> Then you will find – it's your own affair
> But you've given your heart to a dog to tear.

Already, after so short a time together, I felt Butch gets me better than anyone and, unlike the people who surround me, had no great expectations. Butch was never annoyed or upset at my doddering slow progress. He never told me I should take it easy when I desperately needed to feel as engaged with life and work as ever and, whilst he was sad when I left for the office or the shops, his joy was so delirious and uncritical when I came home, he made even the dullest day seem sunny and bright.

The poet, Ruth Padel, once wrote, 'A dog enshrines all your memories – friends, family, self – sixteen years is a lot of history.' After only a couple of months Butch was sharing this difficult part of my history in a more empathetic manner than any of the people around me. My family, used to an active powerhouse of a wife and mother, found my shuffling and slowness a little alarming and, I suspect, rather dull and too burdensome to want to deal with, after the prolonged health problems I'd suffered in the past couple of years. Butch had no such baggage to carry. He accepted me as I was. He had, said David, become my shadow.

It was Ruthie, the physiotherapist, who began to express concern about the lack of progress I was making, despite her best efforts. She had massaged, manipulated and put me through carefully designed paces in the local swimming pool and appeared mystified that, not only was there no improvement, but the symptoms in the right leg were beginning to mirror those in the left. I'd found a pair of crutches that had been lurking around the house since one of the boys had broken his leg. I couldn't manage at all without them. Every step was agony.

It was Ruthie who suggested a call to my surgical oncologist, the consultant who'd dealt with my breast cancer a year earlier, and I knew immediately she too was beginning to wonder if there may be cancer in the bone. I left a message on the mobile of Professor Nigel Bundred, asking him to call me back as soon as he was free. I was on my way to open an art exhibition in London when he called. It was an overblown sense of duty that found me fulfilling an obligation to the organisers, even though I'd been wondering how on earth I was going to manage to stand and make a speech in front of an audience.

I was near hysteria as I described the symptoms to the doctor in detail, explained that I couldn't walk at all without crutches and heard, for the first time in my life, the words 'avascular necrosis'. He couldn't make a diagnosis over the phone, but that was his strong suspicion. He referred me quickly to an orthopaedic surgeon.

Just as I'd had total confidence in Professor Bundred and his ability to employ his scalpel and subsequent medical therapies to try and prevent any recurrence of the little local difficulty in the breast, I now put all my trust in Ashok Paul. He's a short, chubby workaholic of South Indian origin with a no-nonsense bedside manner. But he comes highly recommended. He's the orthopaedic surgeon to Manchester United Football Club, said to have fixed both David Beckham and Wayne Rooney after they'd had broken bones, so I reckoned if he could be trusted with a multi-million-pound footballer's legs, he'd probably be OK for me.

Butch stayed at home whilst David and I made yet another miserable trip to yet another hospital. Mr Paul ordered an MRI scan of the hips. I am ever so slightly claustrophobic and dreaded being placed into the metal tube that feels so like a coffin and makes the most deafening clinking, clanking and grinding noises as it makes images of your insides.

As he looked at the pictures, he had no hesitation in confirming the diagnosis Professor Bundred had guessed at. He explained that the pain I was suffering was caused by deterioration of the femoral head, the ball part of the ball and socket joint that makes the hips work. It is similar to the effects of severe arthritis, but is caused by a disruption to the blood flow to the end of the bone, causing the bone to crumble.

He proffered three possible causes. Maybe I was a diver who'd had the bends. I explained I cant bear to put my face in the water, so I've never even managed snorkelling and when I swim it's like a turtle, arms and legs doing a vigorous breast stroke, head held high away from the surface of the pool. We ruled out diving. Could it be I was an alcoholic? I confessed to liking a glass or three of wine, but wouldn't have called myself addicted. So the booze wasn't the problem. Sometimes it could be a by-product of chemotherapy. Bingo!

The surgeon suggested the least radical treatment which might work if the condition were not too advanced. From the pictures, he thought we may have caught it in time. It would involve drilling a hole into the femur in each leg and might kick start the blood flow. At that stage the sheer torture of walking was so great I would have agreed to anything.

It was March when I went into the hospital for the operation. It would require a general anaesthetic and a couple of days stay. Butch sat on the side of the bed as I packed my bag, pulling things out when my back was turned. He never tore or destroyed anything throughout his puppyhood, but he obviously had the nous to know a packed bag meant going away and he did everything he could either to stop me leaving or, at least, slow down the departure.

He licked my hand as I stroked him 'Goodbye' and slunk off to the sheepskin rug in front of the Aga, looking as woebegone as it's possible for a dog to look. He seemed to know that this parting was to be more than a few hours, or even overnight. I was full of the apprehension that precedes any surgical procedure. It's only natural to worry that you might never come round from the anaesthetic, and I went back to give him another hug, trying hard to stop myself thinking this little bundle of love had just come into my life and I might never see him again. The expression 'hang dog' was invented for the demeanour of both of us.

I've grown to loathe hospitals in recent years after first my mother, then my father, then I had long and painful encounters with a medical profession we'd barely bumped into during a lifetime. Apart from childbearing, the occasional bout of flu or a bit of backache we had all enjoyed incredibly rude health, but deterioration and death had been the hallmark of every passing day for nearly a decade, coming, over-whelmingly, all at once. I suppose it's one of the reasons Butch had been such a welcome addition to the family. The injection of his glowing vigour had been such a relief and a seeming indication that the bad times were all over. But here I was again, dreading the clinical smell, the fearful expressions on the faces of patients and families alike and the anticipation of pain and discomfort. Happily it hasn't spoilt my enjoy-ment of my favourite TV programmes – *Casualty* and *Holby City* – although I definitely prefer my dealings with the NHS to be fictional rather than factual.

The anaesthetist turned out to be a bit of a wag. He insisted on a little chat before putting me out of my misery.

'Mr Paul tells me you present a radio programme.'

I explained that, yes, whilst I was being treated under our family name, I work as Jenni Murray and the programme I present is *Woman's Hour*.

He was unaccountably excited by this news. 'Oh my God,' he squeaked, 'would you mind terribly if I told my wife I'd anaesthetised Jenni Murray?'

I told him I didn't mind a bit and wondered what jokes would be going around his colleagues when he told them he managed to shut Jenni Murray up for a few hours. 'Say what you like,' I mumbled, 'just keep me asleep and alive.'

I have absolutely no understanding of how people pluck up the courage to have cosmetic surgery that isn't really necessary, given how terrifying and danger-ous an experience going to theatre is. I remember coming round in intensive care, wearing tight white stockings to prevent blood clots and feeling absolutely ghastly, with my sons and husband looking down anxiously. I asked them to leave the radio on when they went home, and the first news I heard was that the film director Anthony Minghella had died under an anaesthetic whilst having a small lump removed from his neck. He was a couple of years younger than me. Not something to be fooled around with.

I expected immediate improvement. I was disap-pointed. Mr Paul was encouraging. If the blood flow did get going, the bone would improve. I would have to wait for six months before he could make a judgement and he would need to see me pretty regularly in the meantime. David's attempts at hilarity led to his assessment that 'he's just gone in with his Black and Decker', a comment I later relayed to Mr Paul, again trying to keep my own sense of humour intact. He, with a slightly tight smile, agreed that that was effectively what he'd done, although the equipment was perhaps a little more sophisticated than I'd implied!

Butch, wisely, made no observation, but was pleased to be brought, secretly, to visit. Now I could really see the advantage of a dog that was small enough to fit into a pocket. He peeked out of David's coat, sniffing and smiling, but seeming to know he'd be in the most dreadful trouble if he tried to jump out or leap on to my legs. He brought no grapes and no flowers, just his little, adoring, cheery self. I tickled his ears and could not have had a more welcome visitor. David explained that he was inconsolable in the house. He moped around the kitchen, where, of course, under David's regime, he had to spend the nights, and even seemed to be off his food.

Uncharitably, I wondered for a moment if he was only missing me because I was the one who catered to his every desire for comfort and cuddles. The meltingly adoring look in his eyes convinced me. He was missing his soulmate – just as I was. I couldn't wait to get home and back to my dog.

After the requisite two days' rest I could get about on crutches, but the standard metal ones provided in hospital are heavy and ugly. I spotted a woman who'd had hip replacements trolling off down the ward on a purple pair and learned from the nurse that they were 'designer crutches' made in Germany and could be found on the internet. Apparently, I discovered later from a young man who'd wrecked his leg during a skiing trip, that they are standard issue in France, where even disability is chic! I ordered a black pair. At least if I was going to be a cripple, I'd be a stylish cripple.

When I was finally released, Butch was there in the car to greet me. He sat patiently on the back seat as I lowered myself gingerly on to the passenger side and then, very carefully – no intemperate leaping involved – crawled between the seats and up on to my lap, curling up with a contented sigh, whilst studiously avoiding the site of the drilling at the side of each thigh. I marvelled at how intuitive he seemed to be about my pain and discomfort and felt an immediate sense of relief as David drove away, anxiety about the future etched on his face, that at least one member of the family was unconditionally overjoyed that I was back.

At home, we were back to the same old routine, except now he did the stairs ahead of me, galloping up, two steps at a time, and waiting patiently at the top for me.

There was a phone call from Mr Paul's secretary before my first appointment – a couple of weeks after the surgery. I was quite looking forward to seeing him, having an X-ray and seeing if there'd been any improvement. I was also quite keen to show off the small weight loss I'd achieved – something he'd advised might help the hips. It hadn't been easy. What can be more depressing than being stuck at home, barely able to walk and eating nothing but protein, fruit and veg, just when you need the comfort of bread and chocolates?

He couldn't see me at the next visit. He would be away for six weeks. Would I like to wait until his return, or see another consultant? I opted for another consultant. It seemed unwise to go without a check-up and I tried to pump her as to why Mr Paul had to be away for so long. Was he ill? Had he had an accident? Mr Paul's secretary was trained in absolute secrecy and gave nothing away.

The new guy confirmed my suspicion that there seemed to be no improvement at all and that, in fact, if anything, there seemed to be some deterioration on the right side. My heart fell to the flat-heeled, clumpy boots my condition had forced me into wearing and I fought back the tears of frustration, even though I could have told him things were getting worse without the X-ray. I could feel the ball grinding in the socket with every step, but had hoped against hope that he might have more encouraging news. He recommended that I see Mr Paul on his return and plan the next stage. I left his consulting room as despondent as I've ever been, with no hope of speedy recovery and getting back to being my old, active self.

Meanwhile, I was beginning to learn what it was to be disabled. There was one early morning at *Woman's Hour* where, just before eight, I had to do a trail to advertise what we had coming up in the *Today* programme. I stood up from the chair, grabbed hold of the crutches, and couldn't move. I'd seized up completely. We knew there was a wheelchair somewhere in the building, but we had no idea where it was, so Clare, the producer, plonked me back into the typing chair and wheeled me at top speed along the corridor to the studio. There's a hump – probably some sort of draught excluder – at the entrance. She practically gave herself a hernia trying to heave me over it. Somehow we managed and the job got done and we laughed about it. But it's humiliating, after such a long time of being in complete control professionally, suddenly to find oneself dependent on the kindness of others to complete the simplest of tasks.

At Macclesfield Station there's a lift from one platform to the other. Each journey taking me from home to London involved wriggling out of the taxi which brought me from home, being helped into the wheelchair by one of the lovely station staff, wheeled to the door of the train and then being encouraged to haul myself somehow on to the train. At Euston the little blue buggy with the flashing light and irritating klaxon came to the train to pick me up. Sometimes it turned up on time, sometimes it didn't and you were left sitting on the train hoping the guard would come along and make a phone call on your behalf. There are obviously not enough such buggies to cover the number of people who need them, and the staff are overworked. And if you haven't remembered to book disability assistance at least 24 hours in advance there is no chance of getting one at all. Again I felt helpless and old beyond my years.

Eventually the six weeks of Mr Paul's absence were over and I was relieved to be seeing him again. I had total trust in his abilities, despite the lack of progress, although I found his rather cool detachment – typical of the busy orthopaedic surgeon – a little off-putting. There had been no real emotional connection – quite different from the way I felt about my oncologist who knows exactly how to balance intimacy and distance when discussing such delicate subjects as the removal and reconstruction of a breast. Mr Paul had so far given the impression of being a quite brilliant craftsman, but his bedside manner could have been a little warmer.

This time his demeanour was quite different. He looked thinner, paler and his dark eyes, with slight rings of tiredness around them, looked directly into mine, something I didn't remember him doing on earlier visits – he'd always been a direct-gaze avoider. He said he didn't really need to ask how I was doing as he could see from my dependence on the sticks and the strain in my eyes that all was not well. He wondered how I was managing with my weekly commute to London and back. He knew I'd kept going to work as he'd been at home rather a lot and he'd been listening. Ah ha! My cue to ask questions. How had he been? What happened? His response was one of the most impressive euphemisms I've ever encountered,

'Oh, it was a cardiac incident.'

'And I suppose that's code for a heart attack.'

He nodded, guiltily, like a naughty schoolboy who'd been caught out smoking behind the bike sheds. Then he launched into a rant that fell between fury and heartbreak, saying how much he loathed cardiac surgeons because they all look tall, fit and skinny, like racing demons, and he now understood how ghastly it is for a patient when a doctor says you must take better care of yourself, work less hard and lose weight.

'After all,' he looked at me approvingly, 'you know how difficult it is – although I think you're doing very well, you're looking much thinner, and it will definitely help me do my job better and aid recovery if we have to replace those hips, but, you know what it's like. Like you, I have a family who depend on me to bring in the income. And, like you, I love the work I do. And I enjoy my food.' I suspect he has a wife at home who cooks wonderfully.

I reminded him that as far as I was concerned they were the five most dreaded words in the English language. 'You really must lose weight – from a doctor, serious stuff – and that I had initially found him coldly bossy. I had, I said, had every confidence in his ability to drag me safely into the hip op generation, but frankly, when it came to imperious orders on the plumpness front I didn't think when he was lecturing me that he had a leg to stand on, although I hadn't said so at the time because I'd found his manner rather intimidating.

Suddenly we were partners in crime. 'It's so tough, isn't it?' he agreed. 'I mean, what pleasure is there in going home after a long, hard day at work if you can't enjoy your food?'

My sentiments exactly, and my tough little surgeon had been transformed by the experience of being a patient. I told him I thought he would now become an even better doctor as a result of his illness. He now scored ten out of ten on bedside manner as well as surgical skills.

During a long chat we discovered we share a birthday, 12 May, although he is ten years younger than me. Irritating when people with power over you are so much younger, I find. Nevertheless, whilst neither of us had any real confidence in what the stars might determine, we recognised certain shared quali-ties that we fancied may be attributable to our birth date – an immoderate liking for good food and hard work being top of the list.

And so we met, every month, to check on each other's progress. At each consultation I begged him to get on with a hip replacement. Each time I pleaded he insisted he would not perform so serious and radical an operation as a prophylactic measure. I assured him I needed it. He continued to hope that after six months there would be enough improvement in the blood flow to render it unnecessary.

We continued to bemoan our joint tendency to yo-yo up and down, our shared delight in and total inability to resist any sticky toffee, chocolate or treacle sponge pudding and a loathing of exercise of any description.

On one occasion he beamed with delight and couldn't wait to share a new discovery. 'Have you heard of Power Plate?' he asked. 'It's an exercise machine that you just stand on three times a week for fifteen minutes, and it shakes you fit and thin. Even we could manage that.' I told him I feared he may be a little over-optimistic. Nothing could ever be that easy. I assured him I'd give it a go, as it was what the doctor had ordered, but I thought I'd wait until the six months – post drilling – were up and we knew where we were going with the hips. I wasn't sure it was wise to try a machine that may well be perfect for a dicky heart, but I thought, given the shaking, might be absolutely dreadful for grinding hip joints. He conceded the point.

And so Butch and I spent as much of the spring and summer as possible in the garden. I hobbled through the door and leant on the crutches for the short walk to the swing seat from where I could direct his games. He was growing into a perfectly conformed, handsome little Chihuahua. The roly-poly puppy fat was falling off, his ears had begun to stand smartly on end and his antics were endlessly cheering. He'd learned that, given a mistress who spent most of her time at work or lying or sitting down, exercise was best carried out alone without her walking alongside.

Now the weather was warm, the ground firm and the rain rare, he had no qualms about being outside. He proved to be a brilliant retriever – fetching a ball or pulling on a long piece of rope he found hidden in a corner and encouraging me to throw it. He teased Black Cat and Snooker, who seemed to find him as entertaining as I did, and every so often he just raced round and round the flowerbeds as fast as he could, stopping occasionally to sniff the flowers and then leaping on to my lap for a rest.

I longed to be able to take him for long walks when he stood and gazed wonderingly at the fields that surround the house, obviously dying to go off and explore, but apparently too aware of what a good dog is supposed to do – not wander off alone – to indulge his curiosity.

Mr Paul was not having a wonderful time on the Power Plate. It was not as undemanding, it seemed, as he anticipated. On one of my visits I gave him my advice. Just what the patient ordered. 'Get a dog.'

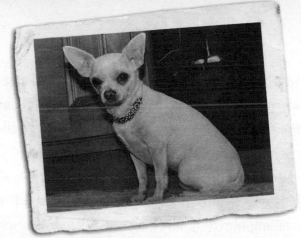

Chapter Five

Hip Op

There was a chill coming into the air as summer drew to a close. The six months since the drilling procedure had almost passed and nothing much had changed on the what-I-could-and-couldn't-do front. I could still crawl up and down the stairs – suggestions of a Stannah Stairlift had been dismissed and the person who suggested it only just lived to see another day – and I had resisted all temptation to have my bed moved downstairs.

My little chum still couldn't come with me to London. I had enough trouble getting myself on and off the trains without worrying about Butch falling down the gap. And David reported a very down-in-the-mouth dog during my weekly absences, even though it was only for two nights and David had been taking him for a few long walks across the fields. Butch had, I was informed, top-notch endurance and liked to roll in cowpats.

I told this story to people who saw his picture – the screensaver on my phone (Is this wrong? Most people have their children.) – and trotted out the usual, 'Well, Jenni Murray, I never saw you as the owner of a yappy rat on a string.' The cowpat story and the long walks somehow gave him greater credibility as a 'proper dog', but I knew I had to stack up the evidence so that I could be more convincing about the fact that he doesn't yap, he barks and is in fact a most attentive early warning system. In other words, a proper guard dog.

I remember years ago, when I worked in local radio, interviewing a reformed, self-confessed house burglar who, during the course of the interview, came out with the classic line, 'You know if it wasn't for the social stigma, I really enjoy the job.' But his relevant comment on the subject of dogs was that any dog was a far better deterrent than any kind of alarm system.

Any alarm, he claimed, could be 'knocked on the head' by a professional crook. A thief might just risk a big dog – they could often be persuaded to quieten down with a tasty titbit – but, he claimed, no burglar in his right mind would tackle the smallest of dogs. They were, he said, noisy, protective, persistent and, if they got hold of you, they tended not to let go.

Butch is ridiculously friendly to anyone who comes to the house invited – even the postman, whom he now knows well and finds adorable, but, even though we joke that he's so kind-hearted he'd probably hold the candle for an intruder, we know from his reaction to any uninvited stranger that he'd die before he'd let them threaten us.

We live in a part of the country which is so remote that we often find walkers passing close to the back door, using the public footpath that's been long established there. Butch has now got used to them and gives them no hassle as long as they stick to the path. But the guy who climbed over the wall into the garden, thinking open access meant he was free to roam wherever he wanted, very nearly lost his leg as a furious little white tornado flew at him, teeth bared. If ramblers come to the door saying they're lost he practically spits, 'You can't read a map?' and sees them off. I've been thinking about a Beware of the Dog sign on the gate!

I spent more and more time at the computer researching the breed's history, determined to add whatever information I could to his defence as a 'proper' dog when challenged. It's not possible to be certain of the origin of the Chihuahua, but, as the name suggests, it's generally agreed they hail from Mexico. The Toltecs, a tribe conquered by the Aztecs, had a companion dog known as a Techichi, the remains of which have been traced back to the ninth century. The skeletons of a dog only slightly larger than the average Chihuahua have been found in the Great Pyramid of Cholula, in the ruins of Chichen Iza in the Yucatan Peninsula. Historical records are said to show the dog was used for hunting in packs.

It's believed the smaller size of the modern Chihuahua may have been brought about by the importation by the Spanish of miniaturised Chinese dogs and cross-breeding with the Techichi. It's also thought to be where the Chihuahua got his bark. The Techichi was mute. It's not a problem that Butch, unquestionably the noisiest dog in the country when he feels his space is being invaded, has inherited to any degree. A progenitor of the smaller dog was, apparently, found in 1850 in ruins near Casas Grandes in the Mexican state of Chihuahua and a letter from Columbus to the King of Spain refers to the development of a tiny dog.

The books describe the modern Chihuahua, first recognised by the American Kennel Club in 1904, as a brave, affectionate animal that tends to bond with one human being, has a clannish dislike of any breed but his own and a tendency to shiver when excited or stressed. I passed this information on to David, who still insisted he needed a coat for his trips outdoors. Not cold at all, just buzzing with the thrill of living.

They are, I was pleased to read, long lived – anything from 14 to 18 years – and their only drawbacks are manic courage out of all proportion to their size (I would discover later, when we faced the wide world together, that he thinks he's a Rottweiler and will happily take one on) and a phenomenon called a molera where, in the young animal, the skull at the top of the head has not joined in the middle, so care has to be taken that they don't bang themselves on the head. Also, the book says, they are picky eaters.

This is far from the case with Butch. He eats whatever is put in front of him, as fast as he can, and always sits at my feet whilst I eat, hoping for a titbit. I save him a little something for when I've finished my meal, and there's nothing he refuses. Meat, vegetables, bread and fruit all go down in record time – he's particularly fond of sweet satsumas and bananas. Only raisins and chocolates are banned as they're dangerous to all dogs, and I don't give him any bones as his throat is relatively small and I'm afraid of choking. Chicken bones, of course, should never be given to any dog as they can splinter in the stomach with disastrous consequences.

As word got around that I was crippled, I began to hear of other people who'd had the same condition after a bout of chemotherapy. One old friend had been treated for throat cancer, another like me had the problem in her breast, and a number of listeners to *Woman's Hour* emailed to describe exactly the same experience. All, in the end, had their damaged hips replaced.

I wish I'd known more about the possible side effects before my symptoms began. The problem in the hips might have been diagnosed earlier and the drilling operation might just have worked. I'm a great believer in information equalling power and, whenever possible, being forewarned and fore-armed. I would have preferred to have been prepared.

The months to September had passed with ponder-ous slowness. If anything, the degree of my disability had increased. I measured out every step from bedroom to bathroom, sitting room to kitchen, back door to car, continuing to refuse to abandon the stairs and sleep downstairs and getting heartily sick of the crutches – smart as they were – and crawling on hands and knees.

Finally, I went to see Mr Paul, the orthopaedic surgeon, at the end of August. We engaged in our usual banter. I was thinking of making a programme about surgery and what it takes to cut into the most precious parts of a person day after day, knowing that you will make them better or even save their life, but will also be committing a kind of grievous bodily harm. He told me he was taught at medical school something which he passes on to his own students.

A surgeon must have the eyes of a hawk, the heart of a lion and the touch of the gentlest of women. 'Great stuff,' said I. 'Now when will you apply all those to sorting out my bloody hips and get me back to being able to get on and off a train and walk my dog … which means more exercise, more weight loss!' (Frankly our slimming and fitness campaign hadn't been going brilliantly for either of us.)

Another scan confirmed that I was not being a wimp and complaining unnecessarily. Mr Paul conceded defeat, the drilling had had no effect whatsoever, and we set a date for a bilateral hip replacement. Usually a surgeon will do one hip and then the other at a later date, because, where the cause is arthritis, one generally gets worse before the other. In my case the deterioration in the quality of the femoral head was fast, relentless and equally bad on each side. As I was relatively young, strong and otherwise healthy, we agreed to replace both hips on 11 September. As the controller of Radio 4, Mark Damazer, pointed out rather wryly, 9/11 was not the most auspicious of days, but it was a Thursday – Mr Paul's operating day – and the earliest date he could manage. I couldn't wait.

I expected to be scared. I wasn't. Perhaps I'd become more blasé about surgery after a mastectomy, reconstruction of the breast and the earlier drilling attempt, or maybe I just felt if something went wrong that death would be a welcome release from the relentless agony. There comes a point when everything you've ever held dear about yourself – your fitness, your independence, your elegance – seems simply to have been washed away, and it comes as no surprise to me at all that for those who suffer constant pain – which no safe painkiller can touch – and the loss of their sense of self, suicide can seem the only option. Or the thought of just sliding into sleep on the operating table and never having to wake up and face the tough demands of recovery appears rather attractive.

I expected there'd be a lot of pain in the immediate post-operative period and I was dreading having to get off my bed and walk, but everyone I'd spoken to who'd been through a hip replacement had said it gave them back their life. I gritted my teeth and endured the epidural – an unpleasant procedure where anaesthetic is injected into the spine, often as pain relief during childbirth, but, in this case, designed to relax the legs whilst they're detached from the hip and re-attached with a metal prosthesis, ease some of the post-operative pain and discomfort and prevent any movement in the first 24 hours. A little prick in the hand followed, and I slid off happily into fully anaesthetised sleep.

I'd considered staying awake. The novelist Maeve Binchy had told me a wonderful story of how she'd had one of her hips replaced with an epidural and what she described as happy pills and said she'd had a jolly time, cracking jokes and making the theatre staff laugh. She'd had none of the grogginess that anaesthesia leaves you with. My surgeon wasn't keen. It would take several hours to complete both sides and I suspect he couldn't face the prospect of me acting as if I were the host at a gruesome party.

I came round lying on my back with a wedge between my knees and registered the dire warnings that I must on no account attempt to cross my legs – a surefire way of dislocating the surgeon's handi-work. I vaguely recall anxious sons and husband at my bedside and not much more for 24 hours, although I do remember vivid dreams involving me and a little white dog storming across the fields surrounding our home. Wish fulfilment indeed.

And then the terrible shock of two smiling physio-therapists standing at my bedside with a Zimmer frame and an uncompromising order that I should get up. The mere idea seemed quite ridiculous. I still had legs, but I wasn't sure they belonged to me. They insisted, and carefully I slid sideways across the bed, swung the feet to the floor and stood up. I suffered no pain, but suspected the morphine might have something to do with that, and listened carefully to the physios' instructions.

I was not allowed to cross my legs for at least eight weeks. I couldn't sit on anything that was low slung. It would be dangerous to make anything more than a right angle at hip level for the same period. I wasn't forced to walk that first day, but it seemed a miracle that I could stand and sit. The new joint took my weight and allowed me to bend enough to sit down relatively easily on the high hospital bed without that sense of bone grinding on bone. It seemed miraculous.

One day later I was making tentative steps into the corridor, shuffling along with my Zimmer frame like a tired, stiff old lady, but the progress was rapid and every day I could go a little further. After three or four days I got rid of the hated Zimmer and took up the fancy crutches again. It was time to attempt the stairs. One step at a time, slowly, slowly. I wouldn't be allowed home until I could make it using the banister on one side and a crutch on the other on my own. It felt insecure and I was terrified of falling, but, apart from feeling a little sore around the huge wound on each side of my body – I had to sleep on my back – the pain I'd lived with for so long had gone. In less than a week I was saying goodbye to the ward staff, armed with instructions on how to exercise, a reminder that I must not sit in a low chair for at least six weeks for fear of dislocation and a clear command not to go back to work for 12 weeks.

Butch was waiting patiently in the car and leaped about in happiness as I approached the door. I couldn't have felt more joy than I did at his cheery little face being there to greet me, and I was tremendously grateful to David for having taken on not only my care, but that of Butch too, even though he'd had such early doubts about the wisdom of owning another dog. I was thrilled too that, despite his awful anxiety about getting me safely into the car, driving me home and looking after me again, he'd taken the trouble to include Butch in our reunion. David understood how much Butch meant to me and to my recovery and seemed not to mind at all that Butch made no bones about where his first love and loyalty lay – with me.

There was a cushion on the passenger seat to increase the height, and I slid gingerly across, behind first, and lifted my legs into the car with my hands. I hadn't yet the strength to lift them independently. Butch peeked through the gap between the two front seats, sniffing my arm and reaching down to lick my hand. He made no attempt to leap on to my lap. How did he know how to take such pains with me?

It took a while to gain the confidence to abandon the crutches and move to a stick, and the 12 weeks were pretty much up and I was ready to return to work when I finally plucked up the courage to walk without any reassuring support, but the results of the operation were truly wonderful. The pain had simply vanished. The greatest joy was taking short walks around the garden, up the drive and back, across the flattest of the fields with Butch at my side. He would run like a mad thing away and back, stopping just short of my feet, demonstrating yet again that there is an intuitive understanding between us. He knew he had to be careful not to trip me up.

Then it was Butch's turn to submit himself to the surgeon's knife. Whilst David was reluctant to have

William castrated, this time he listened carefully to Ed's advice. It is a strange experience when your child overtakes you in his knowledge and expertise. But, as a vet, he argued, he really thought the best thing was to do it. It would not change Butch's personality, but it would reduce any risk of his wandering off in search of any bitch on heat. As far as Ed is concerned, it is the sign of a responsible dog owner to ensure their animal is not sowing his wild oats where they are not wanted.

I held him on my lap as we drove to the surgery. A tall, highly professional young man, dressed in surgical greens, approached with a consent form to be signed, took Butch from my arms – he looked so trusting and I almost dragged him back – but Butch knew the young man well – after all, he is family – and settled happily in Ed's embrace. I was reassured that I shouldn't worry, Butch would be well looked after and Ed would bring him home himself at the end of the day.

I couldn't help thinking that this was my kid – how could I possibly trust him to do something so serious as operating on my dog? But I watched them

disappear towards the operating theatre and, despite
everything I know about the horrors of being wheeled
into the theatre, I would honestly have preferred it to
be myself. Butch seemed so tiny and so fragile. I
could hardly bear the thought of him being anxious
or hurt. My fingers and toes were crossed all day –
but not the legs, of course.

At lunchtime I called and he'd come through
the operation OK, but he was still sleepy from the
anaesthetic. At six o'clock I heard the door opening.
I was having a rest in bed and Ed pounded up the
stairs. He lowered Butch gently on to the bed, and
he marched up to my chest and licked my cheek.
I'm forgiven, then. Ed warned he might be a little
groggy for a while and shouldn't be allowed to run
around or jump on or off the furniture for a day or
two.

At which point Butch leaped from the bed, ran
across the bedroom, picked up his favourite toy, ran
back to the bed and leaped up to me again, asking me
to throw it for him to fetch. I took the vet's advice
and encouraged Butch to lie down and have a rest.
He conceded, but had clearly proved that he wouldn't

obey the doctor's orders and felt absolutely fine, even though he might not be so Butch after all.

Generally I hate having to take time off work, although sharing my sick bed with my little companion made it considerably more amusing than it otherwise might have been. Until the breast cancer incident I had always prided myself on never having been absent in more than 30 years. Indeed, the only programme I had ever missed came as a result of a sudden attack of laryngitis of which I was totally unaware until I actually got to the office. It was whilst we were still in London and I would get up in the morning before the rest of the family for my 7 o'clock start. I got into the car, drove to Broadcasting House without speaking to anyone and it was only when I tried to say good morning to the producer and nothing came out that I realised I wouldn't be able to perform as I had no voice. Dilly Barlow came in, I wrote the script for her and gave her the low down on the research, and the next day I was back and OK.

This time, though, I found I was really rather enjoying the time at home – partly, I think, because I dreaded going back to the weekly commute and was nervous about getting on and off trains with the new hips. They still felt a little as if they didn't quite belong to me. But it was mainly because being at home with my dog constantly at my side had been such a pleasure for both of us and I knew I still wouldn't be quite ready to have him with me on those long journeys to London and back. I had to learn to look after myself properly before I could take full responsibility for looking after him.

There was also a further setback. It was a cold night, as winter had begun to set in, when Butch and I were alone in the house. We were sitting cosily in a comfy chair, him curled up on my lap, when the fire began to falter. It needed a dose of coal to form a good basis and then a couple of logs. A sensible person would have used a small shovel to load on the coal. I picked up the scuttle, swung it around and felt something go. I'd had it before.

I should have known that I had to take care of my back, especially when everything was so weakened by the constant onslaught of medical procedures. I had started going to Pilates classes, so my intentions were excellent, and whilst I couldn't get up and down from the floor without holding on to a chair to steady me I felt as though I were progressing and could feel the muscles getting stronger all the time.

But there was a weakness in my lower back from years of riding horses and the last time I'd felt this sharp pain was when I had a fight with a typing chair at the office which suddenly sank without warning. The usual solution was to go to the osteopath, who put one leg across the other, made a big click and all was well.

Off I went, bent almost double, expecting to walk out of the treatment room upright and fixed. The osteopath was sorry, but it was not an option so soon after the new hips. Fear of dislocation again. He tried to stretch it back into place, practically lifting my head from my body, but it had no effect. If anything, it made it worse.

I suffered dreadful sciatica, a searing pain which zips from the spine, through the buttock and down the back of the leg. Friends at the Christie Cancer Hospital, where I'd had my mastectomy and for whom I now do charity work to raise funds, recommended one of the pain specialists, who took me in for a series of steroid injections which have to be done as a day patient, but in a theatre. I was beginning to think I would go mad if I ever again had to see the inside of a hospital and could only hope the jabs wouldn't have other unwanted side effects. They helped, but didn't entirely cure the problem.

I'm certain my breast cancer was the result of hormone replacement therapy, and once you start these invasive and vicious treatments you enter a cycle of dependency where one problem is dealt with, but knocks on into another. And we are helpless, too afraid to say no to something like chemotherapy – which I'm sure in 100 years' time we'll look back on as barbaric – because we're told it may help save our lives.

A friend at work recommended a cranial osteopath whom she describes as having magic fingers. I was becoming desperate to get moving again. I lived with an entirely rational fear of having to become dependent on a wheelchair, and decided, yet again, to put my trust in someone who might be able to help.

There was no clicking or cracking, but she placed her hands under my spine, did gentle manipulation and I felt the strange sensation of fluid moving around.

She explained that it works by stimulating the spinal fluids that carry messages from the brain. I can't honestly say I really understood enough about how the human body functions fully to comprehend what she did, but after each visit I stood a little straighter, bent a little easier and walked a little less like a penguin. I was active and mobile again and feeling somewhat better disposed towards the mysterious wonders of both ancient and modern science. I began to think I could plan to take my canine companion with me on my next trip to London.

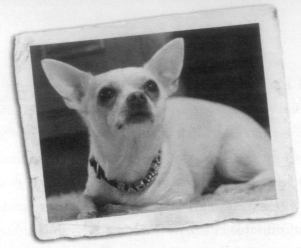

Chapter Six

Virgin Traveller

The biggest of big days arrived. Our journeys together were to begin, and Butch followed me around the house as I made my preparations without his usual hangdog 'oh no, she's leaving me again' look. His sensitive antennae had picked up a different atmosphere and he seemed excited with anticipation.

The hips were working as well as could be expected without any support from crutches or stick and I was able to climb on and off the train to London and back with the minimum of assistance. The staff at Macclesfield Station still stood by the door to make sure I got away safely. They could not have been kinder or more helpful. At Euston, which still felt as daunting as Mount Everest, I continued to use the disabled buggies to get me from the platform to the taxi. I regretted every youthful, energetic, snidey moment I looked with disdain at people who couldn't 'even manage to get themselves to the train'. It's taken such a short time for me to become one of them.

Butch and I had had a lot of help with our preparations. Kate Leigh is our most supportive friend and my ally and backstop in all matters canine. She's a retired midwife who lives alone with a small gang of her own dogs. They're an unusual breed called Bolognese – white, fluffy and small – all of whom, despite their size, make Butch look like a mouse.

Kate's house is a rescue centre for any Bolly in need of a home or just a period of TLC. She'll also take a friend's dogs in for holidays or even an overnight stay, and Butch goes to stay with her if we have to go away for a weekend or short holiday where we have to be dog free. She adores him almost as much as I do and he gets on famously with her brood.

This is a rare occurrence, as I was frequently to experience as we became more mobile. He generally dislikes any other dog he encounters, and Kate tells scary tales of her walks in the woods with the pack when Butch becomes the protector of the whole group. A police officer exercising his Alsatian had been his most recent adversary. The Alsatian, apparently and happily, backed away nervously. We do worry, though, about how little understanding he has of his own diminutive stature. He may not always be so lucky.

There had been little progress in my attempts to adapt Butch to walking on a lead, partly because we'd barely ventured beyond the garden and fields at home and, whilst in the past I'd been a firm trainer of the dogs I've owned, Butch seemed to be able to wind me around his little paw at every turn. When he'd spun around in protest at being constrained I'd taken pity and let him run free. And I hadn't made any attempt, as he grew out of his puppy settling-in stage, to insist he move into his own bed. I'd got quite used to snuggling up against my hairy hot water bottle.

I suspect Kate is every bit as soft when it comes to sleeping arrangements during his short stays with her. In fact, I know for certain he had been as insistent about crawling into her bed as he was into mine. But she had been stricter about walking discipline. Perhaps it had helped that he had been in the presence of her well-behaved animals, but he had now become the model of correct behaviour when his lead was attached, trotting along nicely at my side as I rocked along, still imitating the gait of a rather plump penguin.

On Kate's advice I had bought him a harness. It's blue (I know, I shouldn't fall into this colour stereotype, but the only alternative is pink and, honestly, could a dog called Butch really be seen out in pink?) The harness is soft and pliable. It goes over his head, around his front paws, clasps under his tummy and clings comfortably to his contours. Kate's theory is that he feels more secure with the lead attached to the harness than he did with it pulling on his collar, and it certainly makes us feel safer. If anything untoward should happen whilst we're out – say an encounter with an unfriendly stranger – he can quickly be whisked up into my arms without strangling him.

He detests having it put on. He seems to dislike the feeling of having something pulled over his face and leads me a merry dance whenever it appears. 'Come on,' I say in my most encouraging tone, 'let's put your coat on.' He sidles towards me, his eyes bleeding suspicion. As I bend over to pick him up, he leaps out of the way and stands, guiltily, just beyond my reach. I try offering treats to lure him closer, but he's wise to that one and stays at a distance, silently imploring me not to make him wear it. This goes on for five or ten minutes as my tone becomes less and less coaxing and more and more threatening.

It's a war of attrition and eventually he lets out a deep sigh of resignation and lets me grab him. On with the harness as his nose curls in disgust. It covers up his 'Bad Boy' rhinestone collar. I'm not sure I want all and sundry to see the rather camp neckwear, which I find hilarious but am reluctant to allow the rest of the world to witness. Butch, rhinestone, Bad Boy – bit on the weird side if you think about it.

On with his lightweight chain leash and we were ready for the off. He adapted to travelling as easily as if he were Sir Ranulph Fiennes. We trotted down the drive – well, he trotted, I tottered, towards the waiting taxi. Bag in first, then I slid on to the back seat, still somewhat gingerly, and he jumped in and sat at my feet. He knows he's not allowed to sit on my lap when I'm wearing work clothes. I developed a fondness for black trousers and tops some years ago as a kind of anti-fashion statement. It makes life so much easier not to have to make tough decisions about what to wear every morning and I simply jazz them up with a colourful scarf thrown over one shoulder, the scarf helping to conceal the slightly skew-whiff results of the mastectomy. Black garments and a white short-haired dog who moults profusely at certain times of year, despite my efforts with shampoo and brush, are not a good mix, but somehow Butch seems to understand that his mistress can't look smart if she's smothered in white dog hairs. He's a clever little chap.

He sat patiently at my feet whilst I tried to answer the driver's curious questions about how he's going to cope with getting on the train and enduring the nearly two-hour journey to London. I had absolutely no idea and was beginning to think it was one of my more lunatic ideas. He seemed so tiny and vulnerable to be exposed to such a big wide world.

His first appearance at the station caused quite a stir. He was quickly the centre of everyone's attention. If I heard 'Aww, he's so sweet' once, I heard it a million times and he patiently endured petting and patting from adults and children alike – looking ever so slightly miffed as anxious mothers asked, 'Does he bite?' He gave them a disdainful look. 'As if,' he appeared to be saying and gave excited infants a reassuring lick.

He had to learn the routine. Over first to the ticket machine. Sit quietly and guard my bag whilst I fumble with wallet, credit card and phone where the codes are written in an email. I dealt with the machine – in with the card, type out the code, wait for the tickets to drop and remember to take out the card – whilst he gazed around us, unfazed by the dozens of people who come and go.

Next is the little shop where we buy our copy of the *Guardian*. Again, he sat quietly at my side. And then, the moment I was dreading: on to the platform, where the trains can whizz past at tremendous speed, making the kind of noise one would expect to terrify a small animal.

We made our way through. We had to walk along Platform 1 and take the lift to the other side. Suddenly he stopped. He wouldn't go forward. He tried to wriggle his way to my right side. He was on the left because I was carrying the heavy bag on the right. One of the staff came over and laughed.

'You're walking him on the wrong side of the yellow line,' she said. 'He knows he's supposed to be inside it and furthest away from the edge of the platform. I wish all my passengers were like him.'

I moved him over to my right side and readjusted the bag so that we were both walking well within the yellow line. She was right. He now moved along the platform with absolute confidence and when a train arrived and began to slow he paused for a second, assessed that we were both perfectly safe, appeared to have no fear of the size or sound of the locomotive, and we made our way to the lift.

This, I thought, was bound to be trouble. He was going to hate the noisy doors opening and closing and the sense of movement going up and then down over which he had no control. Not a bit of it. He behaved like a slightly bored businessman – smartly dressed, repeating his familiar commute. He walked calmly into the lift. Stood back quietly from the doors as they shut. Waited patiently until they opened again and walked out as if he had been doing it all his life. Over the bridge, then the whole process in reverse without so much as a flicker of fear.

On the opposite platform he stopped until I adjusted his position – from right to left, making sure he was well within the yellow line again – and we walked along to a seat to await the arrival of our train. I would have expected him to be scared of getting on to a train at a terminus station where, at least, the train has been stationary. I fully anticipated he'd be terrified of mounting a great, noisy beast that had pulled up alongside him and where there was a significant gap between the platform and the first of the steps.

I couldn't have been more wrong. The train stopped. He followed me towards the door marked Coach H. The door swung open. I considered lifting him up, but he seemed so completely unfazed, I decided to see how he would manage jumping up himself. I threw my bag inside, grabbed hold of the bright yellow handle just inside the door and lifted myself on to the first step and then the second. In one phenomenal leap he went straight from the platform to the inside of the train, looked slightly astonished that he'd made it, wobbled a bit as the doors closed and the train began to pull away and then calmly followed me through the compartment door and to our seat.

I took out the sports section of the *Guardian* – the bit I know I'll never read – laid it out carefully on the seat next to mine and lifted him up. He had a quick peek out of the window as the countryside rushed past and then snuggled down to sleep. I felt like the proud parent who's just watched her child successfully complete its first day at school, especially as people passing on their way to the toilet or the buffet car spotted him, stopped, gasped at his beauty and were most effusive about how incredibly well behaved he was. Their dogs, they told me, would never cope with such an ordeal. We both sat quietly preening ourselves.

He politely acknowledged the attentions of the ticket inspector – there's only one, after months of this weekly journey, at whom he barks and he's the one who insists on wearing his hat – rolled over appreciatively for the cooing women who bring the coffee and cold drinks and perked up immediately when the sandwiches came round. I never give him food until I've eaten first.

Pack behaviour dictates that the leader eats their fill before anyone else is allowed to tuck in, and Butch willingly accepts he's the underdog, just staring at me longingly until he gets what my father always called, for some reason known to no one, even himself, his 'gnawpins'. It's a strange word for the little bits of treats you place on the side of your plate to feed to your dog when you're done and I've never been able to find its origin.

Butch merrily gobbles cheese and pickle, egg and cress, beef and mustard, followed by a portion of orange or banana. And then, satisfied, off to sleep again until he hears the guard announce we're about to arrive at Euston Station. On this first trip he stretched himself ostentatiously, jumped down from his seat and followed me off the train – another big leap down to the platform and he hopped, entirely unfazed, on to the waiting buggy. He stood on the floor of the vehicle, gazing, as we 'beep beeped' our way from the platform, across the concourse and out to the waiting car, in astonished fascination at the hustle and bustle of one of the world's busiest railway stations. He was amazing.

We arrived by taxi at Wuthering Depths. There's a metal staircase from the ground to the basement and, after a thrilling sniff around the lamppost outside the gate – unfamiliar territory to a country bumpkin like Butch – we took ourselves along the path towards the steps. Here, for the first time since we left home, there were signs of trepidation. He was fine with a roaring locomotive and two or three feet from platform to train, but a short, open, metal staircase almost defeated him. He stood at the top looking extremely suspicious. I went down a couple of steps and said, 'Come on,' in my sweetest and most encouraging tones. Still he stood, four square at the top, not daring to jump down. I climbed up again, stroked his head and agreed to give him a hand. I lifted him carefully down on to the first step. He shivered, took in one huge breath as if screwing his courage to the sticking point and made his own way down the rest behind me.

I opened the front door and he stepped, a little gingerly, into this new territory. I took off his harness and lead and he stood just inside the doorway, mystified as to what we were up to, and began to make the distressed little mewling sound that generally means 'Quick, I need a pee.' The one great advantage of the flat is that it has a huge, 100-foot garden. He followed me through the sitting room and along the corridor towards the kitchen and I opened the back door. He flew out, delighted to familiarise himself with a safe outdoor space, did what he needed to and ran happily back indoors.

He was relieved to discover there were dishes in the kitchen which had food and water – just like at home – had a nibble and then set out to explore. He raced around the sitting room – checking out the warmth emanating from the gas fire and testing out each sofa and chair to see which was the most comfy and which of the throws offered the best opportunity for snuggling under. Chihuahuas are natural burrowers and like nothing more than to be snuggled under anything that will offer a cosy bolt hole – a duvet, a cover or a cushion will do, although the preferred option is to dive under your sweater if you've offered your lap.

Next came the bedroom. He jumped on to the bed and began to test out the ease of lifting the pillow end of the duvet for future reference. For this he stood lengthways by the bedhead and pushed his nose over and over again under the end of the duvet until he'd found an easy access point. Having established that all was well and there was plenty of comfort to be had, he emerged and spotted the little row of soft toys that have sat on the bedhead ever since the children were small and used to come and stay with me on workdays during the school holidays.

Butch's fondness for soft toys is boundless. They are not for cuddling or snuggling – I serve that purpose to his entire satisfaction – they are for fighting, sometimes, rather disgracefully, despite the operation which unmanned him, for pleasuring himself and, eventually, for killing. His choice was a grey elephant with enormous ears and a trunk and for the next half hour he raced around the flat throwing it into the air, growling at it and tearing it much as a lion would attack a defeated antelope. By the end of playtime one ear was in one corner of the sitting room, the other was on the sofa and a copious trail of white, fluffy stuffing was scattered everywhere.

I spent ten minutes picking it up and throwing it away, as I'd done so many times before with the dozens of snakes, teddies, lambs and monkeys he'd torn to shreds over the past months. The only toy I haven't bought is one that has a squeaker in it – I couldn't stand the noise and I long for someone to invent a soft toy that has some sort of stuffing that can't be ripped out and thrown everywhere.

I really can't complain. He rips his own things to shreds, but he's never touched a shoe or a sock or a garment or a piece of furniture. He has a sure instinct about what's his and what belongs to other people – a very unusual and fortunate trait in any young dog.

Eventually we snuggle up on the sofa and watch crap TV together. Unlike other more discerning members of the family he's entirely uncritical of my fondness for my favourite programmes – on this particular evening it was *EastEnders* and *Holby City*. Generally, to those who criticise, I argue that, in my job, I need to keep abreast of popular culture for research purposes. The great joy of being with Butch is that I can indulge any shameful pleasure because he really doesn't care what I do, as long as I do it with him.

He was delighted to discover that what we do in this strange place is much the same as what we do at home. Something to eat and drink, a bit of telly or a book, quick nip out to the garden last thing at night and then bedtime. He had now become so used to the routine he was tucked up in bed whilst I was still in the bathroom brushing my teeth. I joined him, gave him a cuddle, read for a little while and turned out the light as we both drifted off to the strains of late-night Radio 4. We are creatures of habit.

The early morning had a strict routine too. Should I get up in the middle of the night to go to the loo, he had learned there was no point in bothering to rouse himself. He used to jump up and follow me, my permanent shadow. Now he knew the difference between a temporary and a long departure and simply stayed curled up, knowing when I would be back and when I wouldn't. But when the alarm goes off at six on a work day he knows very well it's up quick and get on with it.

He waited patiently on the edge of the bed as I staggered bleary-eyed around the bedroom, dragging on a dressing gown and making my way to the door. I opened it and he dashed out and dashed back as quickly as possible. Even on balmy mornings he prefers to be indoors with me. If it's cold or wet he can't be out and in fast enough. He waited by my feet whilst I opened the pack of moist food he has in the morning – half a packet each day – and gobbled it in his usual greedy manner.

I put down a bowl of fresh water which he rarely drinks and a bowl of dried meat and biscuits which he nibbles at as the day progresses. He then stood outside the shower as I began to get myself ready for work. He still found it astonishing that I choose to get wet all over every morning and gave me the now familiar 'poor, deluded fool' look.

He followed me back to the bedroom and sat on the bed, watching the curious ritual of drying the hair, slathering cream all over the face, poking oneself in the eye with a pencil, rubbing a brush all over the cheeks and turning pink, then the struggle to get the bra done up, pants and trousers pulled on, and I know he wonders how on earth I can bear to pull something over my head every day with no apparent ill effects.

Duly spruced, I slipped on my shoes and accompanied him out to the garden for a last chance to relieve himself before I got back in a few hours' time. This he found strange. On the occasions I've gone to work when we're at home the ritual has been pretty much the same, but David was around to keep him company and let him out mid-morning.

Nevertheless, he followed me out, rummaged in the undergrowth and followed me back into the flat.

I closed the bedroom door. I didn't really want to risk any accidents in there if he couldn't last out the long morning until I got home around lunchtime. I found his elephant, popped it down in front of him and told him, 'Right, now there's your toy. There's plenty of food and water and you can snuggle up on the sofa. Mummy's (yes, I have gone bonkers) going to work now, so be a good boy and I won't be too long.'

He made as if to follow me to the front door. I told him no, he had to stay behind, and I cannot begin to describe the utterly forlorn and lonely look he gave me. Butch has the most expressive face I've ever encountered in an animal. He can grin and smile with joy when he's happy and he can look more miserable and accusatory if he feels he's being badly done by than I could ever have imagined.

I remember when my first son was small and he would clutch my skirt and beg, 'Please don't go, Mummy,' when I left for work. I felt distressed and guilty for months until his Nanny told me he would then turn around to her, smile and say, 'Right, Jeanne, now what are we going to do.' Butch didn't have the words and he had no company to turn to. He was to be alone in a strange, unfamiliar environment. I felt like the most cruel, heartless woman in the world.

And it didn't get any better as the days and weeks went on. We became familiar faces to the staff on the stations, the trains and the buggies, and his early promise on our first trip was fulfilled week after week. He was the best possible travel companion. But he never got used to being left alone. I began to adjust my lifestyle to accommodate him. I couldn't escape from work, but I refused all invitations to lunch or dinner unless we were both invited, as most restaurants in this country – unlike the French who have a much more relaxed attitude to their canine companions – will not have a dog darken their door.

My favourite and nearest restaurant did allow him to come one evening when a group of friends were meeting for a special occasion, but only on condition we sat at a table away from the rest of the diners and he hid by my side. He, of course, behaved impeccably and was rewarded with a little bowl of his own lamb stew. It was a happy, but a one-off occasion.

Even work was affected. I refused to stay later than lunchtime no matter how persuasively a producer asked me to do something a little extra. I dashed out of the building at lunchtime like a bored clock-watcher, longing to see his joyous little face peering through the curtains. He knew exactly when I was expected and stood in the windowsill waiting for my arrival. And then, every morning, there was the same woeful ritual of the haunting little white figure standing, head bowed, ears forward, in the middle of the sitting room, silently begging me not to leave him. Something had to be done.

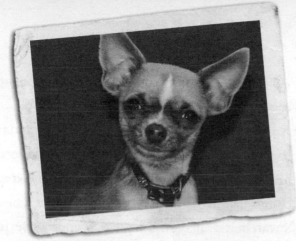

Chapter Seven

Matchmaking

It was quite plain that the only possible solution to Butch's lonesome misery was a companion – someone to play with and cuddle up to when I wasn't available. There was only one problem. David was so reluctant to have one dog, how on earth was he going to respond if I doubled the number? He had, of course, fallen in love with Butch, buying him toys and even a doggy playpen, which had only been used on a couple of occasions, as it took Butch no time at all to learn how to jump out of it. It did, though, provide a backdrop for the dozens of photos and videos Dave has taken of him and his antics. He was so besotted, he even made a website called Butch-theChihuahua.com and posted some of his videos on YouTube! (see the Appendix for YouTube links.)

Nevertheless, he could have presented a serious obstacle. So, working on the time-honoured principle that it's better to apologise than ask permission, I found myself scouring the internet for Chihuahua adverts just as I had previously done to find Butch. I wanted a female, not because I thought breeding would be a good idea, but it seemed obvious that, like William and Mary, a male and female would be most likely to get on well together and be less combative than two males.

It took me several weeks to come up with a possibility. The breeder was in Chester, not too far away. The colour sounded interesting – a kind of caramel hue – and the photos of the puppies were adorable. I called and asked to see them and explained that I was looking for a companion for a dog who was just over a year old and it was obviously important that he accompany me to the viewing as I needed to be certain that he would get on well with any puppy I might buy.

We agreed a time for the visit and, as David was away in Devon on a course, there was no need to tell lies or concoct explanations for Butch and me going off on a trip. We set off early to give us time to find the address as we were not yet technologically advanced enough to have a sat nav. Butch sat quietly on the passenger seat, but seemed to have picked up some of my excited anticipation. If he could talk he'd have been asking, 'Are we nearly there yet?'

We found the house in good time. It was a small terrace on a busy main road on the outskirts of the city. I parked, put a lead on Butch – we'd done the palaver with the harness before setting off – and risked life and limb getting out of the car as traffic rushed by. Butch waited patiently until I opened the passenger door and let him out on the pavement side and we walked smartly to the door, rang the bell and a tall, large, blonde, rather beautiful Russian woman answered and invited us in.

We were ushered into a small sitting room and offered a coffee. There were signs of canine occupation everywhere: toys, chews and blankets, but neither sight nor sound of an actual dog. A long conversation began about how a Russian came to be living in a little house in Chester – she's a tour operator, originally from Moscow, and it's her daughter who breeds the dogs to help finance her studies. I was a bit concerned that I may have come to a breeder who was more interested in the money than the welfare of the animals, but could hardly get up and walk away at this stage of the proceedings.

The daughter arrived. She was in her twenties – also tall and blonde and even more beautiful than her mother, with sharp Slavic features, an exquisite figure and astonishing blue eyes. Her English was perfect and without accent. She introduced herself to Butch, deemed him a fine example of the breed and clearly exceedingly well looked after. I puffed out with pride, but felt I had to explain that he'd been castrated, so I was not looking to breed, but seeking a playful companion. Breeders, I know, can be a little strange if they suspect you may be intending to start your own pedigree line. They like to protect their own business.

'Well, OK,' she smiled, 'shall we let the dogs in?'
I had been beginning to wonder if there were any
dogs at all as we'd heard no sound and, frankly, was
having all kinds of ludicrous fantasy imaginings
about what we might have got ourselves into. The
words Mafia and Russian came unwelcome into my
head!

The house was of the style where the sitting and
dining rooms are divided into two separate areas by
a wall made up of doors which slide open, making
one larger area. The daughter opened the doors and,
I swear, forty-odd Chihuahuas flew towards us. It
felt as though we'd suddenly landed on the set of
Beverley Hills Chihuahua where the little gang of
Mexicans turns up to aid the lost and pampered
Californian with cries of Ne Mas – no more. (It's a
great little film, portraying my favourite breed as
tough little creatures who are determined they will
no longer be seen as spoiled toys to be carried around
in handbags and dressed in designer frocks or shirts
and trousers, exactly the message I'm keen to get
over myself, and curiously unsentimental for
Hollywood.)

Butch was terrified. He'd been sitting silently and politely by my side and he flew on to my lap and then on to the back of the sofa behind my head. The dog who'll take on a Rottweiler obviously knew he was no match for an army of his own kind.

Then, from the mêlée, came one tiny creature. Even at that age, four or five months, she exuded an air of authority. She jumped on to my lap, gave me what could only be construed as a cheeky grin, then she too hopped on to the back of the sofa, sidled up to Butch and licked his face as if to reassure him that all was well. He sighed with relief and the pair of them climbed down on to one of the cushions alongside me and curled up together.

It looked to me like the beginning of a beautiful affair.

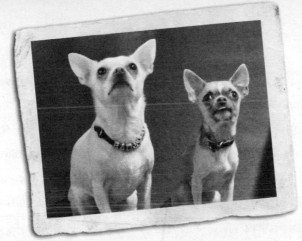

Chapter Eight

Julie

They called her Julie but she was not one of the puppies for sale. I looked at the others, who were sweet and cute, but had none of her character or slightly queer looks. Her face, with its dark, bush-baby rings around the eyes, massive ears, entirely out of proportion to the rest of her, and slightly cockeyed white stripe down her forehead, bore a strong resemblance to the Meercat that says 'Seemples', or Gizmo in the *Gremlins* films or even

Yoda from *Star Wars* – the force was certainly with her.

She was, I was told, an unusual grey colour, known in the trade as Blue and, judging by her size at her age, she was going to be a highly prized 'teacup' Chihuahua. It was intended that she should be used for breeding.

Not only did I love her immediately for the sympathy and rapport she had shown to Butch, but I felt immediately that I was in the hands of some sort of Cruella de Ville – it seemed horribly cruel to plan to breed puppies from something so delicately built and tiny.

The two women spent a lot of time trying to deflect me from 'Julie' and on to the caramel pups. They were ready to leave. They were well socialised. They would have fine conformation. I tried to like them – who couldn't? – they were indisputably sweet and made no objection to being picked up and stroked by a complete stranger and given the once over by a possible suitor.

But Butch wasn't interested, and neither was I. His attention was all on 'Julie' and hers on him, although she occasionally leapt to the floor like an Olympic pole-vaulter and scurried around with her mates – leader of the pack, without a doubt – but always coming back to me for a pet and then to Butch for a smooch.

'I'm really not interested in any of the others,' I said decisively. 'It's this one I want,' pointing at 'Julie', by now curled up again and sleeping with Butch. 'They're obviously a match made in heaven.'

'But, I tell you, she no for sale ... we love her very much ...' The protestations, followed by my insistence on my preference, went on for quite some time and then, at last, came an opening from the daughter. 'Unless ...'

Tough hagglers, these Russians, but I felt the possibility of negotiation coming on and knew, without any doubt, that if I was to have her she was going to cost me, big time.

The owner quoted a price I am not prepared to reveal as, were it to land in the public arena, it may well constitute grounds for divorce. I mentioned a lower figure, to no avail. They were going to have their pound of flesh or no deal. I've never before had to agree a price first stated and have always prided myself on being a pretty tough negotiator, but I was no match for these two. The mother had wrestled 'Julie' from Butch's arms and was clutching her rather too tightly for my or the dog's liking. I feared she might suffocate in the ample bosoms and voluble protestations of utter devotion.

To save her, I took out my cheque book and signed with a flourish.

'There,' I cried, 'the asking price.' The daughter grabbed the cheque and I prepared to take 'Julie' with me.

'No, no, no!' shrieked the mother, most emphatically. 'You no take dog until cheque cleared. We been cheated before. You collect her next week.'

'Then why don't I just give you a substantial deposit and pay the rest on collection? That way we're both reassured there's no cheating,' I suggested.

'No, no, no – we no cheat. Anyhow, you know where we do leev, so you can always find us. We no have any idee from where you are coming ... you pay all or nothing.'

Every sensible bone in my body was saying, 'Don't do it,' but my heart had been won by this little scrap and I had to have her. All the good advice I've been given and have dished out about how to deal with dog breeders was put aside.

We left, despondent, and I spent an entire week wondering and worrying that we'd somehow been caught by organised criminals who made their money out of sentimental English animal lovers. I checked the bank account and the cheque had cleared by the Thursday. On Saturday I had to be at the Hay Literary Festival to talk about my *Memoirs of a Not So Dutiful Daughter*. The best plan was to travel down there by car, taking Butch with me. He would sit angelically through the gig and then we'd drive home via Chester, if all went honestly, taking 'Julie' home and arriving just before David got back from his course in Devon.

On the Friday night Ed and I sat chatting in my bedroom and I could no longer conceal my excitement. He's the vet (sorry, I don't mean to go on about it, but I am his mother!), a great animal lover and I felt sure he'd understand.

'You'll never guess what I'm doing tomorrow,' I grinned.

He took one look at me with that knowing expression from son to mother that says I'm the only person who can actually read your mind and he said, at once, 'You've bought another dog and, Mum, whilst I understand you wanting a companion for Butch, I do hope you've agreed it with Dad, because this is the one thing about you that really hacks Dad off – that you just go ahead and do things without consulting him, and this time you may just have gone too far. He's going to be really pissed off and I really don't want the two of you to split up. Give him a call and at least warn him.'

I sort of knew he was talking sense and was really quite proud that I'd raised such a thoughtful and perceptive son, but I gave him the line about apologising being better than asking permission. I was afraid that, if I called, David would utter a firm no and that would be that. Ed sighed and called me incorrigible and I kept my fingers crossed that I knew my husband better than he did.

The day at Hay went successfully to plan, Butch was undoubtedly the star of the show, sitting like a cherub on the knee of the interviewer throughout my performance and prancing around proudly as people came over to compliment me on the readings and the chit chat, asking me to sign their books and admiring my adorable little dog. But my concentration wasn't really in it. By now it wasn't the money I was worried about. I was terrified of arriving at the house and finding they'd done a bunk and I wouldn't be taking her home.

I rang the bell with some trepidation – still hearing no responsive barking as one would expect from a house full of dogs. If Butch is a classic example of the breed, they're generally the best of guardians of their property. He barks (barks, please note, not whines or squeaks; his voice is deep and undoubtedly manly) at the slightest hint of an intrusion.

Either there was no one there or they had some mysterious trick of making knocks at the door or ringing bells inaudible to animals. Or maybe they were all kept outside in cages and couldn't hear because they were outdoors? Again, I was desperately worried that I'd landed on unscrupulous breeders, although the animals I'd seen on that first visit had all appeared incredibly well cared for and used to being around people.

Finally the door was opened to an effusive welcome and an explanation.

'Ah, you are wondering why you no hear barking dogs. We always keep them in the back of the house when visitors are coming and you no can hear nothing from there. This road is so dangerous and there are so many of them. We are frightened that somehow one of them will escape when door is opened and will run out to the traffic. Please to come inside. Julie is ready for you.'

My sigh of relief must have been audible. Mother smiled and showed us through to the sitting room and offered me a coffee and Butch a bowl of water, which he disdained. He was looking around anxiously, expecting a similar onslaught to the one he experienced last time. It didn't come, but she did, following the daughter from the kitchen as she brought the coffee and a huge plastic bag. 'Julie' has a curious, jiggly gait. Her front paws rise at every step like a trotting horse and her bottom has a definite wiggle. She was just as adorable and characterful as I remembered.

'Julie' jumped on to my lap and renewed her acquaintance with Butch every bit as sweetly as she had before, and he appeared delighted to see her. Mother delved into the bag.

'Now, here you have everything you need. Her own blanket which will carry the scent of her companions. She will not feel lonely. Here is her own teddy bear, enough food for a few days – she should no change her diet, only slowly – her pedigree papers, her vaccination card and insurance for four weeks and her clothes.'

I regarded with undisguised astonishment a generous pile of cotton frocks, hoodies and coats, all in miniature size, beautifully clean and freshly ironed, and wondered how on earth they managed to keep an individual wardrobe for such a vast number of Chihuahuas.

'No, that's fine,' I demurred hastily, 'I really don't think she'll be needing the clothes, although the other things are very kind and thoughtful of you.'

'But she must have clothes,' said mother, her pronunciation emphasising an 'ez' at the end of clothes – clothez – 'she look so pretty in her leetle dresses.'

Now pretty, she's not. I saw her more suited to a hoodie as she definitely has an air of the canine criminal about her – a positively evil look at times – although I had no intention whatever of dressing her up like a doll, be it in pretty frocks or fleecy sweatshirts. But my protestations were useless and we readied ourselves to leave.

Mother and daughter insisted on helping us out to the car, mother clutching 'Julie' to her breast and keening her distress at letting her 'favourite baby leave home'. The bag went in the boot and Butch on to the passenger seat. The, by now, former owners stood guard at the passenger door as I got into the driving side, looking for all the world as if they'd prefer to whisk her back into the house and whispering sweet farewells into her ear in Russian. Their sadness seemed genuine, but, good grief, will she only understand instructions in Russian, will she have to learn a whole new language?

She was placed gently on to the seat next to Butch, the door was closed to much weeping, wailing and exhortations to keep in touch and 'let us know how she go on'. She seemed utterly unfazed by the transition, curled up at Butch's side and, as we pulled away, fell asleep, only waking once when I stopped at a lay-by to give her a private once over away from what had turned out to be an over-emotional parting.

She sat happily in my hand, lighter than Butch had ever been, even at her age. I concluded that he is the rugby prop forward of Chihuahuadom, well built and powerful, whilst she is the Kate Moss, long skinny legs, big ears and acutely conscious of her charms. Her ears stood erect and she was listening carefully with no apparent language barrier.

'OK,' I told her, 'you're not called Julie any more. Your name is Frida – as in Kahlo. Now she was a Mexican artist – and your kind hails from Mexico too. And she often painted herself carrying a little Chihuahua just like you – and, just like you, she was what's known as a *belle laide*, that's French for beautiful and ugly all at the same time, because that's what you are, so there, from now on it's Frida.'

Not sure if she got it, but I was beginning to wonder about my sanity, giving a lesson in the history of art to a dog! She did appear to be understanding every word, and Butch gave me one of his pitying looks. I guess he thought I'd finally lost the plot and gone mad. He could be right because now I had to face the possible wrath of 'him indoors'.

My heart sank as I arrived at home and found that he had got there before me. I'd hoped to be in the house, have the animals settled in and a cup of good strong coffee inside me before having to face the music. Nothing for it but to brave it out and argue it as a case for animal welfare partly brought on by his own insistence that I should be solely responsible for dog care. Which was why I hadn't bothered to mention it. Plus she, like Butch, would be travelling with me to London because Butch needed the company, which was why I'd agreed to have her in the first place, and if I hadn't had her, well, goodness knows what might have happened to her.

I rehearsed the speech before getting out of the car. I emerged with Frida tucked up in my arms and Butch following closely behind. I took the bag out of the boot and headed for the kitchen door. He was sitting at the kitchen table. I dropped the bag on the floor, stitched a smile of welcome on to my face, made for the table, and out of my lips came the following:

'Look, look what I've got. It was soooo sad. One of Kate's friends had a litter, she's quite elderly and this was the last one left and she just couldn't get rid of it, and the old lady just couldn't keep her, so Kate thought of me ... that it might make a good companion for Butch. I hope you don't mind, but I just couldn't resist. Isn't she sweet? Her name's Frida. And she didn't cost anything.'

Oh, wow, what a whoppa! I have never in nearly 30 years together told anything more than the whitest of lies. I quite shocked myself, but secretly patted my own back that I had always dealt with the family finances, because he really couldn't be bothered. I come from a long line of Yorkshire matriarchs who dealt with everything concerning money and had never had to ask their men for something to spend, nor been checked up on. No risk of his finding out that Frida had come far from free! (I have since told the truth, now she's an established and much loved member of the family, so it's not a problem if he reads this, but I was just desperate for him to be pleased, sympathetic and welcoming.)

Which he was. His eyes melted as he took in the tiny little figure who looked up at him so winningly. Right from the start I saw her amazing talent for getting anyone she chooses on her side. And her fondness for men. She had definitely taken to me, but she positively fluttered her eyelashes at first David, then Edward, then Charlie. The boys were, unsurprisingly, joshingly rude about my fondness for 'rats'.

'Crikey, Mum, we thought Butch was bad enough, but this one really does look like a rat. Why don't you get something that actually looks like a dog?'

But it wasn't long before she was hopping from one of their laps to another, ensuring that everyone in the family thought she was the bee's knees. And there was unanimous agreement that the clothing she'd brought with her was unsuitable for any dog, let alone such a feisty little madam. I'm afraid it all went into the bin.

She settled in brilliantly – cuddling up in my bed, just as Butch had, but needing the same, if not more attention to toilet training than he had required. She must have been allowed to get away with anything at her previous home and thought nothing of weeing on the duvet. She only did that the once *chez nous*. My fury at having to strip the bed and cart the duvet off to the laundry knew no bounds. But she had no problem with sloping off into the corner of a room and had to be watched like a hawk, whipped outside every time she moved from a lap and praised profusely when she did it in the right place and roundly bollocked if she didn't. I asked Butch for assistance in teaching her the correct way to behave, but, much as he seemed to enjoy her company, there was a hint of a glint in his eye when she was being ticked off. It hadn't occurred to me that there might be an element of sibling rivalry. I'd had plenty of experience with the boys when they were young and had often accused them, during their fights, of having the worst case of the syndrome since Cain and Abel. I should have known that Butch, the older 'child', would resent the affection showered on his little 'sister'. It was there, peeking through, right from the start, in snidey little snaps from her if he tried to push

her off my knee or out-and-out battles over a favourite toy.

Next came the knotty problem of travelling with
not one, but two Chihuahuas. Frida was so impossibly tiny I couldn't yet find a collar that would fit her
and the smallest harness I'd ordered on the internet
arrived, but swamped her. It was pink – sorry, I know
I shouldn't have fallen again into such obvious sexual
stereotyping, but, as I said, they only came in pink
and blue and they couldn't wear the same, could they?
But I would have to wait until she grew into it. There
was no possibility of taking her on the double lead I'd
planned and it would be far too much to expect her
to leap the great distance from platform to train.

Much against my better judgement, I bought a
special doggy bag. It's black and bears a strong resemblance to a briefcase, with net down the sides and
along the top to allow her to breathe and see where
she's going. She settled down inside it quite happily,
made no fuss about the trip in the taxi, the noise of
the train coming into the station or the movement as
we set off. Once in the carriage, as usual, I laid down
the sports section of the newspaper. Butch took his

place and I lifted her out of the bag to sit next to him. She snuggled up, fell asleep, woke for the titbits when the sandwich lady came around and contentedly drifted off again. Just like Butch, to my great relief, she was a natural traveller, settling in to whatever environment she's faced with and invariably deliriously flirtatious during the endless attention she attracts at the station, on the trains and in the street. Mission Accomplished.

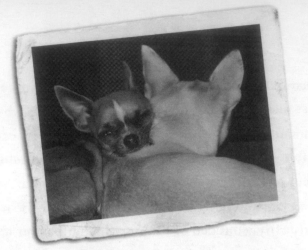

Chapter Nine

One Plus One

I remember a friend telling me, just before my second son was born, that one plus one makes more than two. More than double the work and more than double the worry. Happily my mobility was improving all the time and, although I was stiff as can be first thing in the morning, there's nothing like two wet noses rubbing across your cheek and four appealing eyes gazing into yours to convince you there's no room for a lie in when two hungry, thirsty little creatures are desperate for the toilet, taking in the first fuel of the day and then a good run to expend some of their boundless energy. The warm weather helped the aching limbs and scuttling around after them certainly got me going.

The sibling rivalry did not diminish. I was constantly reminded of the 'me, me, me' palaver that had gone on for years between my two sons – and still does to some degree. I told number one recently that we would be making a shower room in part of his brother's bedroom and got a 'why his room, why not mine?' The fact that they're both in their twenties, can hardly be said to live at home any longer and that the room where the shower was planned was right next to the necessary plumbing seemed not to have occurred. It was sheer favouritism … obviously!

The pair of them – Butch and Frida, that is, not my sons – followed me around everywhere. David called them my gang. Kitchen to sitting room, sitting room to bathroom, bathroom to bedroom. They sat like a pair of bookends waiting for me to finish at the loo, jumped on to the bed for a snooze whilst I sat at my desk to work and both leaped on to my lap as we settled down in the evening to read or watch television. And woe betide me if I dared to pet one and not the other or offered a treat to one without having the other's ready at once. The paws of the ignored one scratched at my knees, crying, 'Me, me, me.' Just like children.

If I had ever thought that girls would be calmer, quieter, less boisterous, less aggressive than boys, Frida overturns every stereotype. Oh, yes, she's a flirt and knows exactly how to use her allure to get whatever she wants, but she's no slouch in the 'pushing-yourself-forward-and-using-brute-force' department if her winning ways don't work. She may be tiny, but her strength and tenacity are formidable. She reminds me of Queen Elizabeth I, with 'the body of a weak and feeble woman, but the heart and stomach of a King!'

Butch did his best to retain his reputation as a gentlemen. He made a point of taking the stairs slowly and carefully to make sure there was no danger of tripping me up. He waited, even at an open door, because he knows a well-mannered dog always lets the pack leader go first. When told to come, he came, immediately. When he was asked to sit, he sat and waited, even when there was a tempting titbit coming. When he was told to find his ball, he scurried around the garden, remembering where he left it last, dropped it at my feet and obeyed the instruction to fetch.

Frida is the most ill-mannered, self-centred and demanding creature imaginable, but impossibly cute and affectionate with it – irresistible. At feeding time she seemed to acknowledge that Butch is top dog and waited whilst his dish was put down first. During her settling-in period she would pick up a chunk of meat and disappear into a corner to eat it in private. Then she'd find her absence had been an open invitation to Butch to scoff hers as well, so she soon learned the best way was to stand firm and eat hers from her dish. She can consume every bit as much as he does, but rather more slowly, and it wasn't long before his attempts to edge her out of the way and finish off for her were met with a growl, then a nip that was intended to hurt. He doesn't even try it any more.

She didn't walk anywhere. She rushed about like
Zola Budd on speed. She took the stairs two at a
time, with no thought for anyone else's safety, and
never walked around any obstacle. She flew over it in
much the same manner a winning horse would take
Becher's Brook in the Grand National. She perfectly
understood 'sit', but would only comply if there was
a rug or a carpet beneath her. Not a chance on the
kitchen tiles: much too cold for her delicate sensi-
bilities. Any open door was an invitation to fly
through it, any order to 'come in, right now' was
read as 'come in when you're ready', and an order to
'fetch the ball' was construed as 'wait till Butch gets
it, then do your best to prevent him from bringing it
to me'.

Her methods were pure evil. She chased after
him, waited till he picked up the ball, nipped his
bottom or his neck and engaged in what looked and
sounded like a vicious fight, at which point he had to
drop the ball in order to defend himself. She tried to
snatch the ball, but couldn't because her mouth wasn't
big enough. Butch grabbed it and hared around the
garden with it, trying to bring it to me, whilst she

chased him as fast as her little legs would carry her. Alternatively, she marched up to him, stamped her front two feet on the floor, spun around a couple of times and crouched in the 'let's play' pose, which for Frida meant 'let's have a scrap'.

Butch engaged enthusiastically in any fight or race she was up for, wrestling with her on the floor, growling, barking and nipping, then chasing her as she set off like a greyhound, dodging any cat or chicken that might inadvertently have got in the way. We have seven chickens. There are two old ladies – Maran/Wellsummer cross – Ena and Annie – who are dark grey, singularly unattractive, but produce the best dark brown eggs with golden yolks I've ever tasted. Then there are the youngsters, pure bred Wellsummers, not yet mature enough for laying, but together they too form their own gang, are allowed free run of the garden and take no nonsense from anyone or anything – and certainly not from two bumptious little dogs. Butch and Frida learned from bitter experience that cats and chickens can inflict real pain with either claws or beaks and are to be avoided at all costs.

Frida, being slighter and lighter, generally came off best. She's fast and wily. If Butch raced her around one of the circular flowerbeds and appeared to be catching her she simply changed direction and turned the tables. I suppose when you're that tiny you have to rely on quick wits and manoeuvrability. She'd barely grown at all and was easily half the size of Butch and light as a feather.

David and I spent hours on fine days sitting in the garden, laughing at their antics and relieved that no long walks for exercise would be necessary as they seemed to manage to exercise themselves perfectly well, stopping off occasionally for a slurp of the chickens' water, keeping a wary eye out for any chicken that might be offended and in pecking mood. Then there'd be an exhausted flop on to someone's lap, a cuddle with each other and then they'd be off again.

I remembered the breeder expressing the concern that Frida, being so wee, might be bullied and hurt by Butch. Not a bit of it; if there was any bullying going on, she was the perpetrator, although they both seemed to emerge from the fiercest of battles miraculously unscathed.

They seem to have an inbuilt timing mechanism. They sat and watched the Birmingham train which precedes ours come and go without moving a muscle. Then, minutes before our train was due to arrive – to my amazement, the service which was rubbish for donkey's years had suddenly improved and could be relied upon to pull in on schedule – they stood up, shook themselves down and looked up at me expectantly as if to say, 'Come on, train's coming.' They appeared to have the senses of a North American Indian tracker – conscious of an approaching sound long before it is apparent to an untrained human ear.

As it came to a standstill, we walked towards the same door we always entered by. I pressed the button to open the door. I put my bag inside, pulled myself up by the handle conveniently placed just inside to assist the less abled and felt the little tug on the lead behind me as they leaped in unison over the gap and the steps and into the train. All safe and sound, so far.

We sat in the same seat, in the same quiet coach, next door to the loo so that it was not too far for us to travel *en route* (they refused to be left alone at the seat, so it was quite a palaver to go to the toilet).

Down went the newspaper, up they jumped and settled down, both waking to the oohs and aahs of passing fellow passengers, the ticket collector and, of course, the staff with the sandwiches and, if it was a later train, hot stew and cheese and biscuits, followed by a banana. They liked to get a taste of everything.

At Euston we waited for the buggy. Even though my walking ability had vastly improved, at the end of a long day and then a two-hour journey getting from the train to the taxi rank still felt like a major expedition. As it arrived we climbed down from the train and into the buggy – the two of them hopping up with ease. It's only a short journey, but they loved it. They stood near the edge, watching the hustle and bustle of the station concourse with absolute fascination.

Unfortunately, on this occasion, they were standing a little too near the edge of the buggy and I didn't have the lead held as short as I should have. A gaggle of schoolgirls went by, spotted the two of them standing there and shrieked, in unison, 'Oh, my Gawd – how cute is that!' I wish I had a pound for every time I've heard that on our travels. On the days that I felt fit enough to walk about, it took me twice as long to get anywhere as it would normally as I heard those words and then, 'Do you mind if I stroke them?' at which point Butch went into supercool 'stroke me if you must' mode and Frida into hyper flirt, spinning around in excitement and rolling over to have her tummy tickled.

This time she made her usual response to the compliment and flew in the direction of her admirers. Butch had no choice but to be dragged from the buggy with her as the girls and I screamed 'stop, stop' to the driver as he forged ahead, trailing the two of them behind the buggy. Their feet were scrabbling around to gain purchase on the ground, to no avail, and they only narrowly avoided being caught in the wheels. I was helpless to do anything as I didn't dare jump off whilst it was still in motion or let go of the lead.

Cue an enormous crowd of anxious commuters and weeping teenage girls picking them up from the floor and crowding around them whilst I, in total panic, tried to get down and check they were unharmed. I felt each of them over carefully from top to toe and, to my great relief, they appeared to be totally unscathed. Butch looked extremely indignant at the undignified humiliation of it all and furious with Frida, blaming her attention-seeking behaviour for the entire incident. Frida, as usual, revelled in the degree of interest she was creating and seemed really rather disappointed when I rescued her and lifted them both carefully back on to the buggy.

Even the driver, who, after months of using his service, I knew quite well and found usually to be the most detached and unmoved of men, came round to pet them and satisfy himself that there were no injuries. I slumped in overwhelming relief and held them tight on my lap – dog hairs on black clothes forgotten. I held back the tears. Not one for public displays of emotion, I couldn't have been closer to sobbing. I could not have borne it if, through my carelessness, my beloved little dogs had come to grief. If, like a cat, small dogs have nine lives, I reckoned they were down to eight and determined to clutch them close when we used the buggies, despite their straining at the leash to watch the busy world go by.

Naturally, when they go on their visits to Kate, the dogsitter, they are absolutely on their best behaviour. She seems to adore them just as much as we do and praises Butch for his gentlemanly demeanour and good manners and spends most of their stay giggling at Frida's attempts to be the perfect lady guest – a task at which she generally fails.

Kate's house is designed to be dog friendly. There are toys, treats, blankets and beds everywhere. Any marking (where a male dog lifts his leg to mark his territory) is cleaned up with no fuss or harsh words, and every animal she encounters seems to trust her on sight. There's a new conservatory with access directly on to the garden, and I wish I'd seen it, but I had left when Frida decided to take one of her flying leaps from the house to the garden and landed in the pond.

Kate fished her out as she struggled in righteous anger, dried her off and found, after that, that she went about a little more sedately. Getting wet is her least favourite occupation. There's never any danger whilst out on a walk that they might decide to go for a swim in a river or a lake. Her accidental dip in the pond seems to have confirmed her determination to avoid it at all costs.

Kate has her own five dogs, but because she also acts as a rescue centre for any Bolognese that needs re-homing and she occasionally takes in other friends' dogs for holidays, there may be a couple of animals there who Butch and Frida are meeting for the first time. Butch shows none of his aggressive tendency when he's there and even Frida has the brains to know you don't mess with strangers who are quite a bit bigger than you.

But all the boys instantly seem to have fallen in love with her, and Archie, one of the more mature of the Bollys, seems particularly enamoured. Thankfully, Kate, as a responsible dog owner, has had all her dogs neutered and will only take similarly sterilised animals in as guests, so there was no danger of any unwanted pregnancy should she unexpectedly come on heat during a visit there.

It took ages for it to happen because vets won't spay a bitch until she's had her first heat. One year old and Frida still had shown no signs of sexual maturity. I crossed all my fingers that it wouldn't begin whilst she was in Kate's care. It would be such a responsibility to make sure she was kept away from any 'live' dogs whilst she took her brood out for their daily constitutional in the woods.

We decided to go away for Christmas to spend the week with Charlie, who was in France, perfecting his French and having a jolly old time in Biarritz. We would have liked to have taken the dogs with us – the French are so much more dog friendly than we are. In this country you get thrown out of the most unlikely places if you have a dog with you. Kate was ejected on one occasion from Help the Aged and I was chucked out of Smiths whilst buying a newspaper and Boots where I was in search of Ibuprofen for a raging headache. When I looked around – it was actually on Euston Station – I reckoned my dogs were cleaner and probably healthier than most of my fellow customers.

Anyway, I hadn't managed to get their passports sorted out – you have to microchip them and have a certificate to say they've been vaccinated against rabies – and I wasn't sure Ryanair would be too welcoming. Eurostar won't carry dogs. The only way they can cross the Channel is in a car on the ferry or the motorail, so they had to stay with Kate.

And sure enough, the minute we left the dogs in Kate's care, it began. By the time we arrived to pick the two of them up it was all over and Kate looked done in. She had managed to keep her away from any interested dogs in the woods, but Frida's carryings on with Kate's boys had been nothing short of disgraceful. If her flirtatious behaviour had been bad before, it had been magnified a millionfold. She had spent the entire week throwing herself at first one, then another, whilst Butch, his Puritan streak coming to the fore, had looked on in mortified disgust at his sister, the shameless hussy.

Kate's boys were most alarmed as we swept her up and prepared to take her home. Happily, Kate has an acute sense of humour and merely expressed her concern at how her lovelorn lads would pine as their hearts were broken at Frida's departure. And they did look very shaky, but, I would argue, a little relieved that she was leaving. Not sure they could stand the strain.

So now, she too had to be neutered. It's obviously a much bigger and more invasive procedure for a female than it is for a male, but Ed advised that Rebecca, one of the vets in his practice, was particularly adept at the job and would manage it with only the smallest incision. I booked her in.

Nothing to eat or drink the night before. Butch was furious. It didn't seem fair to put down food for him and deny her, although I did sneak him a drink before bedtime. I didn't think he would come to any harm from just one night's starvation – he's a pretty stocky little chap. I left him at home when I took her down to the vet. It felt as if she needed my undivided attention. She looked so tiny and vulnerable as I handed her over and I went through another day of desperate anxiety, just as I had with Butch. I do try very hard not to have a favourite and, although Butch will always be my number one, Frida had managed to worm her way almost as powerfully into my affections.

I got the same advice when I went to collect her as I'd had for Butch. 'Keep her quiet. She's still a little dopey from the anaesthetic and may seem a little unwell for twenty-four hours.' They brought her out to me, looking decidedly floppy, and wearing a plastic cone collar around her neck and surrounding her face. She was to wear it for a week. She had three stitches, and Chihuahuas are, apparently, particularly bad at pulling out their stitches and licking the wound, which can, of course, lead to infection. I was to give her antibiotics, bring her back in three days for a check-up and then, in a week, the stitches could be removed.

She looked up at me with what seemed like relief. I knew at once what was going through her mind. 'Ah, here's the mug who does exactly what I want. If I come over all sad, miserable, in pain and unable to eat, she'll have this bloody collar off me in a second.'

I told her I was sorry, but this time I had to obey the doctor's orders and she was to wear it the whole time, yes, even in bed. If she could have thrown herself to the floor and have a tantrum, she would have.

I carried her into the kitchen, checked the wound – very tiny, brilliantly done – popped her on to the floor on her still slightly wobbly little legs and she tottered to her bed in front of the Aga to sleep off the last of the anaesthetic. Butch let her be, understanding,

I think, that she wasn't well and eventually curling up, comfortingly, beside her.

In no time at all she was up and at the food. There was a slight struggle to get her mouth around it, on account of the awful collar. Then a demand to be let out and within seconds they were chasing each other around the garden as if nothing had happened, except that Frida occasionally misjudged the distance between the garden furniture as she scurried around it. The collar kept on catching her out. She hated it and did everything she could, crying, whining, begging, for it to be removed, but I didn't dare risk it.

She responded by being the most awkward animal ever to be fed a medicine – a dislike with which I do have some sympathy, finding it equally unpleasant that I still need to take a daily pill in the attempt to keep any recurrence of the cancer away and, despite the ever-improving strength in my legs, the occasional powerful painkiller.

Her antibiotics were tablets. Her dose was a quarter twice a day. They could not have been smaller. She clamped her jaws shut tightly. I prised them open and pushed the tablet to the back of her tongue.

Time and again she pretended to swallow it and spat it out when she thought I wasn't looking.

If I tried to trick her by mixing it in with food, she carefully ate around it, leaving the tablet at the bottom of the dish. I can only assume enough went in to do the job, as the collar came off and the stitches were taken out at the appointed time with no apparent ill effects, and at last I was certain that such a diminutive frame would never have to go through the rigours of having puppies.

As far as travelling goes, they are both now adept at living in two places at once. Butch, of course, still hates having the harness put on and will stand at a just unreachable distance when I tell him it's time to get his coat on. Frida is much more amenable and there's nothing like praising Frida for being such a good girl to persuade him to hurry over and offer himself for the torture of having the thing dragged over his head.

So, there are benefits to having the two of them, but there are drawbacks too. Two to worry about, two to keep safe and healthy and, whilst the one is generally the most obedient and obliging of dogs, the second should have 'Bad Girl' engraved on her fore-head. Double the trouble was no exaggeration. Indeed, I'd come across it before. Years ago, as a young producer/presenter in local radio in Bristol, I chaired a weekly pets phone-in where owners could call the programme and ask for advice about their animals. The vet, James Alcock, was President of the Royal College of Veterinary Surgeons – a mine of information with a great gift of the gab and terrific sense of humour. He got me through the bizarre series of engagements with a Mrs Burgess from Bristol who was concerned about a toad that was mating in her garden 'the wrong way up'.

My giggles were ill concealed and I was told smartly by the listener that, 'Miss Murray, I can understand you seeing the funny side of this, but it is a most serious issue.' James bailed me out as I fell under the table in hysterics and advised simply letting the toads get on with it. The story went on for several weeks, the longest mating ritual in history I should think, only to end with the sad news that the female toad had died. The entire West Country wept.

Then there was another, clearly elderly woman, with a strong Bristolian accent, who was reluctant to give her name.

'It's a bit embarrassing, I'm afraid.'

James assured her she needn't worry.

'Well, I've just called you about my budgie,' she said, 'Joey, 'is name is, oh, and he's a lovely little chap. He sits in his cage, happy as Larry, and sings his little heart out and eats his seeds and drinks his water. And I bought him a little toy – you know, one of them Kellys that you can roll over and it bounces back up, and he loves it … he goes mad … and, sometimes, he puts his little wings around it and, I'm not sure I should say this on the air, but … I think he masturbates!'

I went under the table again in hysterics and James calmly advised her that she was probably right and he might be bored. Had she thought of buying him a companion? As we never heard from her again, we guessed the solution had worked. Indeed, getting a companion for a solitary animal was often James's answer to questions about antisocial behaviour, and generally we didn't have any complaints.

One morning a call came in from a chap who had a young Siamese cat. He had 'houseproud' written in his tone of voice. 'I just don't know what to do,' he complained. 'I've provided toys and scratching posts, but he will insist on chewing at my plants – and I have a beautiful collection which I've cared for for years. But I love my cat. What am I to do?'

I wasn't surprised when James came up with his usual answer.

'Mmm, it sounds to me as if your cat is bored and lonely when you're out at work. I suggest you get him a companion.'

It was several months before we heard back from the guy, who, mercifully, appeared to have acquired something of a sense of humour in the intervening period.

'I just thought I'd call to tell you I took your advice and the kitten gets on extremely well with her brother ... but ... I thought you should know, I now have two cats eating my precious plants!'

And that was my problem. Double the trouble. A lesson I should have learned long, long ago. Not that I regret bringing Frida into the family. Yes, she creates chaos, but she and Butch adore each other and everyone she meets is bowled over by her joyful, cheeky little personality.

The only snag is, now they both follow me around, dolefully, in the morning as I shower, make up, dress, pick up my bag and say, 'OK, I'm off to work now. Back soon. I won't be late. Be good.'

And *two* sorrowful faces sink into the deepest woe!

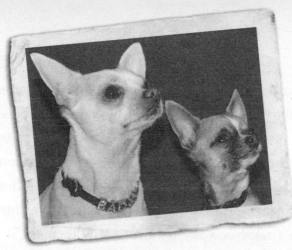

Chapter Ten

Eight Lives Left

It is such a comfort to know I have such a trustworthy holiday home as Kate's – the ultimate doggy
nanny – affordable and reliable! I'd hate to have to
consign them to the discomfort of kennels. I had a
week of long days chairing a conference and then
presenting *Woman's Hour* and going out in the
evening to see plays or films as part of the research
for the programme. Kate agreed to have them from
Sunday to Friday. I would pick them up on the way

back from the Manchester edition of the programme which takes place every Friday.

I arrived home late on Thursday afternoon, exhausted. Much against my better judgement, I acceded to David's insistence when I was ill during chemotherapy after the breast cancer that I should have a television in my bedroom. I'd resisted it for years, despite the boys' astonishment that I believe TV is best as a medium to be watched by an audience and should only be in a room where a family sits down and enjoys it together.

They assumed it was a ploy on my behalf to prevent them from having TV in their rooms, which in part it was, but I really do prefer my bedroom to have nothing but a radio, an iPod for music and lots of books. But I had spent a lot of time in bed during cancer treatment and when the hips were dreadfully painful, and it had been a pleasure to be able to catch up on favourite programmes. I'd been too lazy to take it out when my mobility was better.

I went to bed early, knowing I had to get up at 5.30 in order to get to work on time, but watched the

news and the start of *Question Time*, already beginning to drift off to sleep.

When the phone rang.

'Jenni, it's Kate. I'm really sorry to bother you at
this time of night, but I'm worried about Frida.'

My heart pattered with anxiety.

'She's making a strange choking noise ...'

I tried to reassure Kate that it's a Chihuahua trait.
Occasionally, after violent exercise or if they get
excited, they can sound for a few minutes as if they're
choking as they catch their breath. I urged her not to
worry. I should have known she's far too experienced
a canine carer not to know when something was seriously wrong.

'No, it's different. She really seems to be choking
and coughing and she's been sick. Is it OK if I take
her to my vet?'

I offered to come over, but Kate was insistent that
she could manage and that I needed my sleep for
work the next day. I didn't sleep at all, just waited
anxiously for Kate to call me and tell me what the vet
had said. I couldn't imagine what she could have been
choking on as Kate's house is totally dog safe. She

doesn't allow them, rightly, to chew on sticks, which can be dangerous, and the only toys and chews she has around the place are sold, and presumably approved, as being safe.

Frida, like Butch, has had every prophylactic injection a puppy could possibly need, so she couldn't have picked up any of the diseases such as parvo virus or distemper that could be making her violently sick. I was mystified as to what might be the matter.

It was around midnight when the phone rang again.

'I'm afraid the news isn't good,' cried a desperately concerned Kate. 'My vet has X-rayed her. There is something stuck across her throat. He doesn't have the equipment to remove it because she's so tiny. He thinks she needs to go to the small animal hospital at Liverpool University. So, if it's OK with you, I'll take her there now. My neighbour says he'll come with me so that he can drive and I can nurse her. I'm afraid it's going to be expensive.'

Funny how thought of cost just doesn't occur when a little animal you love is in such desperate need.

'Kate,' I said, 'I'll come right away and take her myself. I can't expect you to be crossing the country in the middle of the night.'

Kate reassured me that she felt it was her responsibility when Frida was in her care; that she'd got her neighbour all set up and ready to go, so they were off. They'd phoned ahead, so they were expected, and I was not to worry. She would be in very good hands. There was nothing I could do. It would take me an hour to get up, dressed and get to Kate's.

I knew only too well what very good hands she would be in, although my anxiety was in no way tempered. I feared she might die *en route* or, if she got there in time, might be too weak to endure a major operation. The vet schools in this country all have hospitals for both large and small animals. The students learn how to work in practice there and the teaching staff are the leading experts in their field. I knew if anyone could save her from choking to death, the university vet school could. I also knew Kate was talking sense about her taking Frida to the hospital. Time was of the essence and she needed to be in expert hands as soon as possible. I thanked Kate for all her efforts and tried to get some rest. As I tossed and turned with worry I resigned myself to the fact that there would be no sleep that night.

Kate called from the hospital to say she'd arrived safely and the staff had suggested I ring in the morning to see how she was doing. As dawn broke I got up to go to work and called the hospital. They tried to reassure me. She was still alive. She had been sedated, the specialist anaesthetist would be there soon and they hoped to be able to remove the offending object by putting an endoscope down her throat. If not, they would have to operate to remove it, but for the moment her life was not threatened.

I spent an anxious morning at work. I jumped to the phone each time it rang, hoping it would be good news and dreading the bad. I never leave my phone on during the programme – it's considered extremely bad form for a mobile to go off during transmission – but I left it on vibrate, not wanting to miss the news whatever the circumstances and battling the pictures in my head of my little, energetic scamp splayed out and expiring on the operating table.

I made my weary way through the programme – no news. The call came from the hospital late in the morning. The operation was a success. A scalpel had not been necessary and the foreign body was removed via her mouth. She was sleeping. She would need to stay in hospital until Sunday. Could we come and pick her up then, perhaps after lunch?

I called Kate to let her know the good news. She was hugely relieved and, like me, whacked out from a sleepless night and worry. Her journey to the hospital had been horrendous. You would think, wouldn't you, that the Liverpool vet school's hospital would be in Liverpool? Kate had been in such a panic the night before, she hadn't checked and had had a dreadful detour when she and her sterling neighbour finally realised, *en route*, that the hospital was in fact somewhere in the wilds of the Wirral, on the opposite side of the Mersey to the city.

I, of course, in my anxiety to check Frida was OK and elicit every detail of her care and her current condition, had forgotten to ask what the source of the trouble was ... we would remain in ignorance until I picked her up. I could only thank Kate for everything she'd done and then start to worry about the cost.

I know from Ed's stories that these highly qualified centres of excellence tend to cost an arm and a leg. He's often referred difficult cases to Liverpool and come home to say how relieved the owners were that their animal was insured.

Now, paperwork is not one of my strong points. I have a pile of papers on my desk which is laughingly known as my filing system. It was this very 'filing system' that, four years earlier, had led to me missing the mammogram I'd been called for and which would have alerted me to the cancer sooner and when it was much smaller than when I finally detected it myself. I'd noted the date, seen it was a day on which I'd be busy, made a mental note to phone up for another appointment, put the invitation on the pile and promptly forgotten about it. If I'd remembered to make that appointment I may well have needed less radical surgery than I had and could have escaped the horrors of chemotherapy. I hadn't learned my lesson from that experience.

On this self-same pile, in fact at the very top, was the insurance certificate that covers Butch – there to remind me, indeed on my list of things to do for that very afternoon, that I must call the insurance company and add Frida to the policy. Truly the road to hell is paved with the best of intentions. I didn't dare ask on the phone what the whole episode was going to cost me. There are certain circumstances where forewarned is not forearmed, just fore excessively worried. I decided to take a cheque book when we went to collect her, make sure Dave was distracted when the axe fell and deal with the awful news when it had to be faced.

Butch has the most extraordinarily expressive face. I've never seen an animal whose feelings and moods can be read in the way his can. When I called at Kate's to pick him up, he was sitting quietly in a corner, his forehead furrowed and his eyes downcast. Even his greeting, usually effusive, was subdued and he was showing no interest in playing with the other dogs, nor in giving Kate her usual fond farewell. If I'd been the suspicious sort I'd have suspected him of a guilty conscience. Had he been responsible for Frida's misfortune? I put it down to sadness at the absence of his pal.

More calls to the hospital brought ever more encouraging reports. She was eating and playing and would definitely be ready for collection on the Sunday, as arranged. We set off early for the long trek across Cheshire and into the Wirral, feeling more and more admiration for Kate and her neighbour as we realised how far from Liverpool it was and how hard it must have been to find at the dead of night.

A veritable bevy of young nurses and vets came out to greet us, rather reluctant, I think, to see her go. One, a young woman, carrying Frida tenderly in her arms, sang her praises. She had been a very good girl. She'd been going to the toilet outside. (Phew, I'd been worried she might have been doing it in her cage and all my good work on the housetraining front might well have suffered a setback.) And she is *so* friendly, *so* playful and *so* cute. Is she just a puppy?

Again, I had to explain that no, she was now fully grown, a year and a bit old, I'd had her for more than six months, and that yes, she was much smaller than Butch. It seemed surprising that members of the veterinary profession were unaware that, like people, Chihuahuas come in a variety of sizes, and again I trotted out the line I've used so many times when people stop us to express astonishment at the difference in their build. 'Yes, he's the rugby prop forward of Chihuahuadom and she's the Kate Moss.' I should carry a tape recording of it to save my breath.

We enquired as to the reason for the whole incident. It was, apparently, part of a pig's ear that was stuck in her throat and she had been very lucky to survive it. It was, they explained, not an unfamiliar problem to them, and they advised that, even though they are sold, dried, as dog chews, pig's ears can, in fact, be very dangerous and the dog, even animals as large as an Alsatian, doesn't always survive. We were advised never to buy anything for them to chew that doesn't soften and dissolve in saliva and never, ever to let a dog play with a stick.

I couldn't blame Kate for it. I know she had them lying around the house for her dogs to play with, but how was she or I to know that a product specifically sold as a dog chew could possibly be so dangerous as to be life-threatening? When I told Kate later about what the cause had been she was mortified and had a vague memory of how it might have happened. Like me she'd been watching the start of *Question Time* in her bedroom and Butch and Frida were playing on the floor having a game of tug of war with a bit of one of the pig's ears. The only explanation was that Frida, in her usual dogged manner, was so determined to win it for herself that she inhaled and swallowed one great lump.

Except, of course, she didn't manage to swallow it. It just got stuck across her throat, and that's when the symptoms started. All pig's ears have been removed from both our houses and I now understand why Butch seemed so guilty about the whole incident. He obviously thought her departure was his fault. He was very happy, smiley and bouncy when he saw she was well again and about to come home.

I suggested that David pop them both out on to the grass outside the hospital while I asked for the bill and dealt with the damage. No point freaking him out on the financial front. In fact, the cost was not quite as horrendous as I'd anticipated. The young vet asked if she recognised our family name. Was Ed, the vet from the practice in Leek in Staffordshire, our son? I answered in the affirmative and she said he'd made a number of referrals to the hospital, our family name is an unusual one and our address was close to his practice, so she guessed we were related. I think we got mate's rates! Some compensation, at least, for all those costly years of getting him through the training.

Frida, when we finally got her home, was entirely unfazed by the horrors of her experience and rushed around madly, checking out that nothing had changed and tempting Butch into a game and a scrap. We cleared the house of anything that might bring about a repeat performance, went around the garden picking up sticks, and determined that they should be left with no toys at all, except under supervision. Butch was not happy to see his plastic balls and favourite teddies put out of reach, but even plastic can be torn and swallowed and all cuddly toys have stuffing which, given the dogs' propensity for ripping them apart, could easily be inhaled.

I wouldn't say I've become paranoid about their safety, but I do tend to watch them like a hawk. I close the gates at home, even though it's a complete pain every time you drive in and out, to make sure they don't wander out to the road. I keep them company, even on a short trip to the garden, in case, in the middle of the wilds as we are, any passing bird of prey mistakes Frida for a tasty morsel. I only let them out alone when we're in London because the garden there is completely enclosed and I don't recall ever seeing a passing kestrel.

I never leave them alone in the car, even in the coolest weather, in case someone takes a fancy to them and breaks in. I've read so many stories about Chihuahuas and other small dogs being stolen, I'm terrified that they'll somehow disappear. They've filled such a lonely hole in my life, my constant companions, I can't imagine how I would cope if I were to lose them. They're funny, affectionate and full of the kind of energy that tends to diminish with age and illness. They're a daily injection of *joie de vivre*. Without them I would, I fear, be turning, unwillingly but uncontrollably, into a grumpy old woman.

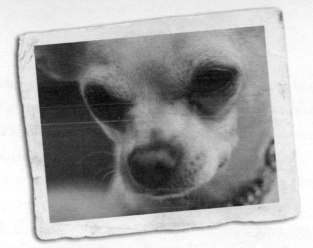

Chapter Eleven

Butch Saves the Day!

Yet again I found myself having to make another demand on the dogs' amazing, nonchalant adaptability. There had been a lot of family changes in the three or four months since the pig's ear incident. Both boys were abroad – Ed traversing the world and paying his way by castrating cats and dogs for charitable institutions across South East Asia, with plans eventually to get a proper job in New Zealand to take him up to the Rugby World Cup in 2011. We've planned a get-together there for the tournament. Charlie was still perfecting his French in Biarritz. It was the perfect time to get the major work done on the house that had been hanging, literally, over our heads for years.

The roof needed replacing, cracks in the stone-work strengthening, the kitchen modernising and the carbon footprint of a house primarily fired by oil and woefully ill-insulated finally improved. The house is listed, so it needed a first-rate, traditional builder and an architect who knows old buildings to supervise the work.

The architect tutted with alarm at the state of the ceiling in my room. There were patches which showed where the rain had found its way in, but it was old and a valuable part of the house, so we hoped to patch and preserve it. But, he warned, careful as the builders would be when they were replacing the roof and getting on with the lagging, there was a remote possibility that the ceiling might come down. He looked anxiously at the evidence that this wasn't simply a sleeping room, but a work room and a library. There were hundreds of books, a desk, a computer and that famous filing system.

'If I were you,' he hazarded, 'I would clear it out completely.' I had no alternative but to move out of the house. The builders assured us the work would take no more than a couple of months. I knew from previous, bitter experience that their calculations would be wildly unrealistic. I needed a quiet place at home in which to work and daren't risk months of hammering, banging and possibly collapse of the ceiling and all the dirt and dust it would bring with it, preventing me from getting on with things.

David and I agreed that I would move into the flat we bought some years ago in Manchester for the nights we couldn't get back home because of being out late, followed by an early morning start, or on account of the threat of bad weather. The snowstorms are not as frequent, nor as terrifying, as they used to be. Our neighbour told us when we first moved into the house that they'd been stuck on their farm in the hills for 14 weeks in 1946. It made the prospect of living there even more attractive to our two small boys who saw a thrilling future of lots of time off school and plenty of sledging ahead. It has never been quite so bad – one or two days off, maybe, but it was useful to have a bolthole in the city when snow or ice was forecast.

I decided to put everything apart from essential clothes, books and computer into storage. David, meanwhile, would remain at the house for site supervision and security. The dogs, naturally, would come with me. I was really not sure how we would cope, on the third floor of a modern block with no garden, but I couldn't bear to leave them behind. Him indoors, maybe, but my babies ... not a chance. Should I be ashamed at being a more dutiful dog owner than a wife? Probably, but David didn't seem to mind too much.

He agreed that they might not be entirely safe with builders coming in and out, perhaps leaving doors and gates open. We packed up the car with essentials and left poor David behind to deal with the imminent chaos with slightly heavy hearts, but a measure of excited anticipation too.

There's a car park underneath our block of flats. Butch and Frida jumped out of the car, quite eager at the prospect of exploring somewhere new – especially somewhere new where the rubbish bins are in the corner and our fellow residents not entirely scrupulous about where they dump their half-eaten pizzas at the end of a drunken night out. Rich pickings for ever-hungry little animals.

We went up in the lift, Butch affecting his usual 'businessman on his way to work' pose and Frida spinning and dancing at the thrill of it all. There's a long carpeted corridor and three sets of fire doors before we get to our front door, but they trotted along like troopers, pausing every so often outside someone else's door from which early evening cooking scents were emanating.

Once inside the flat, they explored every nook and cranny, tried out the balcony, which they didn't like – it seemed to make them feel insecure to be so high up – and sighed with relief when I produced dishes, food, toys and their bed. They settled down with no trouble at all, instantly at home.

It is, of course, an absolute pain to live somewhere that was not designed with dogs in mind. There are no parks nearby, and apart from the pavements there is one patch of rough grass for early-morning and late-night trips to the loo. But they quickly became accustomed to the long walk along the corridor, down in the lift, out the main door, along the little private road to their 'garden', get on with it and then all the way back again. It was fine if there were no interruptions, but it seemed to me I was the only proper grown-up living in the entire building, and encounters with lots of young people were frequent.

There was one young man we saw in the early mornings who took out his very mature, very big and, happily, very calm and patient golden retriever. They lived on the second floor and I noticed, after a while, the dog's owner had taken to using the stairs for his trips up and down, obviously sick of Butch barking and growling at his animal and Frida spinning and flirting like some canine Mata Hari.

Butch never barked at dog-free human inhabitants with whom we shared the lift. He smiled benignly at them, sighing with embarrassment as Frida did her seductive, trouser-scratching me, me, me performance and, as a consequence, got all the attention. Every trip outdoors brought a litany of 'oohs' and 'ahs' and 'how cute is thats'. Young men out with their girlfriends pandered tolerantly to their 'Ooh, can we have one just like it?' only to catch me alone in the lift on another day and demand darkly, 'How many times a day do you have to take them out? Can you leave them on their own? How much do they cost? Can they use a litter tray?' After I regaled them with honest answers I doubt any of the girlfriends got her wish.

Everyone, though, seemed delighted to have them around, apart from the somewhat sour-faced woman from one of the upper floors who clearly detested dogs and groaned loudly if ever we had to share the lift with her and the young Asian girl from the flat opposite who eventually confessed to being terrified of them. It's hard to imagine anyone being scared of anything as incapable of being intimidating as Butch and Frida, but she shook with terror and took the stairs if she spotted us heading in or out of the building. We are, it seems, not a universally dog-loving culture.

We did find a couple of parks we could go to for longer walks. Good for them to get out and vital for keeping my hips moving. It meant a trip in the car and staying on the lead. I was terribly nervous of any encounter with a Rottweiler or pit bull or any group of young men with one of the dangerous breeds of status dog. At least if my two were on the lead I could quickly whisk them up into my arms. Strange that I cared more about their welfare and safety than I did my own. I'm sure a pit bull would have no hesitation in going for me as well.

I did, on one crisp, sunny winter's morning, decide to take them to Heaton Park which I deemed to be relatively safe as it's full of families with young children at the weekends. It's the Manchester park where you're least likely to encounter broken glass on the paths – a terrible hazard in many of the other parks to poor little dogs' paws – and, as they both tugged at the lead to go sniffing in the undergrowth, I decided that, just this once, I'd let them have a good run around.

I was strolling along the path by the lake, there was no one else around and they were having a lovely time investigating leaves and mud and puddles, when a couple of delightfully camp, exquisitely dressed gay guys came around the corner, holding hands and with three Dobermans. They're the kind of dog you see in horror movies guarding the villain's lair: big, black, silky coat, pointed nose and ears, very big teeth. My heart sank. The biggest of the three, obviously an adult male, was straining powerfully at his lead. The two others, young, smaller and, I reckoned, female were running free and made a beeline for Frida. She ran in frenzied circles, squealing in terror as the two bitches chased her, plainly infuriated that one so small could outrun them.

I stood helpless, as terrified as Frida and suppressing a scream whilst shouting, 'Please get your dogs under control,' realising I didn't really have a leg to stand on as mine were far from under control. Each time I tried to grab hold of Frida she evaded my grasp, still running around at breakneck speed with the snarling Dobermans in hot pursuit. I couldn't see how she could escape those bared gnashers.

Butch, meanwhile, ignoring the two females, evidently thought, and I suspect quite rightly, that the real danger came from the angry-looking male and set up the most furious, noisy and intimidating

JENNI MURRAY

performance of a guy defending his girls (me and Frida, I think) – feet planted squarely, hackles raised, teeth bared. The two men had to combine their efforts to hold on to their dog, who responded to Butch with equal fury. Eventually I managed to catch Frida, both of us shaking with fear. The men grabbed hold of their two females as I lunged to take hold of Butch and clip on the leash.

As the guys sashayed passed us, they looked at us with disdainful sneers and muttered loudly enough for me to hear, 'Mmmm, I think that one suffers from small man syndrome,' and continued on their way.

Butch was still snarling with absolute fury and Frida was shivering with terror. After I calmed them down, I couldn't resist a fit of the giggles. The expressions on the faces of those two complete strangers had been so damning, but Butch had shown he was afraid of nothing – to his possible detriment, I fear. Small, he may be, but he has the courage of a lion. Our walks in the park came to an end and we came home as often as possible, partly to cheer David up and partly to give them a chance to run out and be free for a while in the garden and the fields.

And so our weekly trips up and down, to and from London, had to be made from Manchester Station, rather than little Macclesfield with which we are so familiar and where we knew everybody. Manchester Station is huge. We had to familiarise ourselves with another lift as Butch and Frida can't manage the escalator, walk across a vast concourse past Sainsbury's, W.H. Smith's, Starbucks and the like, heading for the ticket machine and, as usual, were stopped every few steps by admiring passers-by. It took for ever and resulted, on one rushed early evening, in the loss of my most important possession: my Blackberry.

I needed it at the ticket machine to get the code for the tickets. As I was juggling two bags, two dogs, wallet, cup of coffee, sandwich, Blackberry and the complexity of the machine itself, you'd think people would have more consideration than to interrupt. But no, a whole group of middle-aged, female dog lovers descended upon us, 'oohing, aahing' and asking the same tired old questions. 'Is she a puppy?' 'Will you mate them?' 'What kind of dogs are they?' I did my best to be polite and patient, but eventually had to say we must go; we had a train to catch.

It was pulling out of the station when I remembered to reach into my bag to switch off the Blackberry. I like to sit in the Quiet Coach where you can get on with reading without being harassed by other passengers yelling, 'Are you there? Can you hear me? I'm on the train,' into their own mobile phones. It wasn't in my bag. It wasn't in my pocket. I panicked. It had all my contact numbers in it and emails from producers at work giving me details of what we would be discussing in the following morning's programme. It had all my favourite photos of my boys and my babies (canine ones, that is). It is truly my life-support system.

In desperation I asked a man sitting opposite if he had a phone I could borrow. I called David at home.

'Oh, hi,' he laughed, 'I thought you'd lost your mobile.'

Good grief, is he a mind reader?

'I just had a call from a guy at Manchester Station. He says he found your mobile on the ticket machine – you idiot – he found this number under "Home" in your contacts list. He says he's taken it to Lost Property. You can get it when you come back.'

Never has a woman been so relieved. He didn't leave his name, so I couldn't call him to thank him, but he definitely restored my faith in the goodness of human nature – a faith that was somewhat undermined when I got back to the station on the Thursday afternoon – two whole days without it had been purgatory – and hurried to Lost Property, where the young, rather sullen man in charge brought it out, unharmed, and charged me £10 for the privilege. It would have been £20 if it had been a laptop. A great incentive not to be so careless or preoccupied again.

The flat was cold when we arrived in London. It doesn't have the benefit of central heating. It's probably saved me a fortune in energy bills over the years, but it was most unwelcoming on a chilly, damp March night.

We flung on the gas fire and the electric blanket and decided the best policy was early to bed, as early to rise is what we do on working mornings. We snuggled up together under the warm duvet and I turned off the electric blanket. No point in having it on all night when there are two little, live hot water bottles to keep you warm and cosy.

When we awoke, all seemed well and as normal. Our routine is to get up at six, a quick trip out to the garden for Butch and Frida and back in for breakfast. They're so used to the ritual, after a couple of years of living together, they now pop back to bed; as I shower, do my hair, make up and dress, they keep a weather eye on my activities, still apparently mystified as to why it takes a person such a ridiculously long time to get themselves ready to go out. They get up when I'm ready to leave, nip out to the garden again for a run around, follow me through the flat, looking morose as I say my goodbyes, and jump on to the sofa to peek through the window to see me off. They're there again when I come back, anticipating my arrival long before I get there.

You remember I said the London garden is so safe and secure I've never worried about letting them go out there by themselves? This chilly, dark March morning was no different. I opened the back door. It was murky and cold, but it wasn't raining so they ran out without hesitation. I turned to go to the kitchen and began to prepare their breakfast when the most horrific noise set up outside. It was the kind of terrified screaming you'd expect from a child who had been injured. I knew it was Frida, and it was joined by Butch barking his loudest and fiercest. I ran – if you can describe my crab-like scurry as running – to the door.

They were flying towards me, Frida first, little legs pounding like pistons, Butch behind her, still growling, barking, snarling and turning his head, trying to escape while at the same time intimidating the dark shape that hunted them down.

The fox, a shadowy and mangy, thin creature, teeth bared, turned tail and ran away when it saw me. I slammed the door shut and turned to the two shocked and petrified little creatures who stood shaking on the mat by my feet. Blood poured from Frida's head and neck. I gently felt her all over. She screamed as I touched her flank. Butch was unharmed, but still shivering with terror.

It was obvious the fox had taken Frida's head into its mouth and bitten down on the top and bottom of her head. The blood flow showed no indication of any damage to an artery, but she must have been shaken and battered because her ribs and stomach were painful to the touch. I disinfected a piece of cloth and tried, gently, to wipe away the blood and the stink of fox breath on her. Butch jumped on to the sofa beside us and did his best to lick her better. The three of us sat and sobbed.

Luckily the small animal hospital at the vet school where Ed was trained is not far away. In the waiting room we learned that a kitten had been killed by a fox in the same street earlier in the week. Frida was found to be severely traumatised, unsurprisingly, but not too seriously hurt, and very lucky that the bites on her throat had not been deeper and that her neck had not been broken in the tussle. It was generally agreed that, had Butch not been there to surprise the fox and defend her, she would almost certainly have been killed. I could not have been more proud of my little hero, putting his own safety at risk to save his companion.

No one in the council seemed interested in doing anything to help, and only one pest control company

I called deals with foxes. They offered to put a trap in the garden which would need to be checked every day. If a fox took the bait, they would come and take the animal away and shoot it. Frankly, the way I felt at the time, I would quite happily have shot the thing myself, but decided to try a less radical method.

My neighbour, Rosie, who lives upstairs and has a dog of her own, volunteered to help with spraying the entire garden with fox repellent. It has to be done across several days and I would only be around for part of the week. I'm not sure it's helped, as other people say they've seen foxes in their own gardens since then, and on one evening, lounging and watching television in the sitting room, which looks out on to the front garden, a bright red, bushy-tailed creature strolled across and paused to look down disdainfully at the three of us. Butch flew at the window and barked furiously, Frida burrowed under my sweater and the fox calmly hopped over the wall into next door's garden.

All of this happened, of course, a couple of months before the fox attacks on twin babies sleeping in their cots in North London and reports of other people who had found urban foxes rather more ready to have a go at the human population than even the animal experts had believed possible.

It seems to me quite extraordinary that the couple whose babies were mauled received hate mail from animal activists after five foxes were reported to have been shot as a result of the attack. Their letters trotted out the sad old mantra of the animal liberationists that an animal's life is as valuable as a human one, so the foxes should be left to do their worst. I wonder what their response would be to the fox that killed the cute little kitten or the sweet and vulnerable Chihuahua?

When I expressed my personal loathing of the fox in the newsletter I write for the *Woman's Hour* website, criticising Roald Dahl for his portrayal of *Fantastic Mr Fox* and describing the animal as the serial killer of the animal kingdom after our entire flock of chickens was murdered one night at home (not Ena and Annie and their crew, but an earlier flock we had when the children were small), I received a number of emails criticising me for my 'prejudice' and arguing that foxes only kill to feed themselves and their young.

The fox apologists should have come out with my children who tended those chickens and went out to pick up their eggs every morning. They found a scene of carnage to compare with a medieval battle-field – blood, feathers and ripped carcasses every-where. It seemed to me the fox had killed for fun, not just for food. The attacks on Frida, the dead kitten or the two poor children I doubt were a result of hunger either. Urban foxes are not short of a bite to eat. I now storm around London in a fury at the number of people who drop the remains of their burgers and chips on the pavements, leave their bins open to the elements or, heaven forfend, encourage the wretched animals into the city by putting out food especially for them.

Of course, the consequences of the attack on Frida continue. Her physical wounds have healed and within two or three weeks she had her mojo back – as bouncy and friendly as ever and not at all nervous on her trips out in Manchester or, now we're back home, in the garden and the fields there.

In London, though, both of them are constantly on edge. In the flat their ears are pricked for every sound, and where, before the attack, they were calm and laid back unless someone came to the door or pounded down the stairs above us particularly loudly, now they run to doors and windows barking furiously at sounds and scents I can neither hear nor smell. They are in a constant state of defence of their territory.

When it's time to go out to the garden they gather at the back door like troops about to go into battle. They seem to know instinctively that attack is probably the best line of defence. Frida especially scratches frenziedly at the door. As it opens, despite my warnings to wait for me to go first, the two of them fly out as fast as their little legs can carry them, barking and rushing around, peering under bushes, around the shed and right up to the back wall, making sure the coast is clear with me scurrying along behind them.

This behaviour has not endeared us to the neighbours. The young couple next door, whose bedroom looks out over my garden, have made numerous complaints. There's very little I can do. I have to let the dogs out early in the morning and last thing at night and there are enough nerve-racking dogs around any inner city to make me nervous of taking them for walks in the park or even around the streets. It's no fantasy to fear a deadly assault from a big dog. An old friend in Bristol was out on the downs there with her beloved, tiny Griffon when a marauding Alsatian went on the attack. Her dog was killed.

There are, as this sadly indicates, disadvantages to owning such small dogs, and a state of near permanent nervous anxiety seems to be my lot these days. Nevertheless, I would not change them for the world. As with my children, I continue to try very hard not to have a favourite. I love them both dearly and cherish those comforting evenings when they both snuggle on to my lap whilst I read or watch television, or they dig down under the duvet for a night's rest or leap and laugh in greeting, tails wagging wildly, when I arrive home.

But, whilst Frida is affectionate, needy, a great time-waster and frequently hilarious (we spent an hour yesterday playing sit for treats and laughed through the whole time as we tested her willingness – or otherwise – to sit on the cold kitchen floor; she now simply heads for the mat when she feels a 'sit' coming on and plonks herself down expectantly), it's Butch who truly has my heart.

He does everything he can, always, to please me. He was with me through the worst of my pain and disability, a constant reminder that there is life after grief and suffering. He's encouraged me to take steps I would otherwise have feared and avoided, leaving me with no excuse just to loaf around and wallow in a kind of Victorian, sofa-bound malaise.

Never have I been looked at by such openly adoring eyes. No dog I've ever owned has ever wanted to be in my company all the time, with no desire to wander off to investigate pastures new alone. He listens to me, follows me, does his utmost to protect me and appears to anticipate and empathise with my every mood playful and energetic when I'm happy and snuggly, considerate and compassionate when I'm low.

I think, if this is not too anthropomorphic and sentimental, that he loves me too. He's my hero, my protector and my best friend, small as he is. It's not, as they say, the size of the dog in the fight that matters, but the size of the fight in the dog. He is, and I hope will be for a very long time to come, My Boy Butch.

Appendix

YouTube links

Butch's website is at:

http://www.ButchtheChihuahua.com

On YouTube, if you search for 'Butch the Chihuahua'
you will find the following links:

BUTCH THE CHIHUAHUA:
http://www.youtube.com/watch?vffi6VbR-AiEWlk

BUTCH THE BRAVE:
http://www.youtube.com/
watch?vffi4Xww_qmWq8g

WHO'S THE BOSS:
http://www.youtube.com/watch?vffizJlfE1H8JUE

BUTCH:
http://www.youtube.com/
watch?vffiToOuzHKDDC8

NODDING OFF:
http://www.youtube.com/watch?vffi6TixmHxmvKA